YOUR WELLBEING REVAMP

A Practical Guide to Thriving in Life and Work

(How, When You Don't Know How)

Séamus Ruane

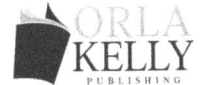

978-1-917728-05-8

Copyright © Séamus Ruane 2025

All rights reserved.

All intellectual property rights, including copyright, design rights, and publishing rights, rest with the author. No part of this book may be reproduced or transmitted in any way, including any written, electronic, recording, or photocopying, without written permission of the author. The content of this book is for informational purposes only and is not intended to diagnose, treat, cure, or prevent any condition or disease. You understand that this book is not intended as a substitute for consultation with a licensed practitioner. Views expressed are the author's own based on their experience as a certified positive psychology practitioner and community pharmacist. Published in Ireland by Orla Kelly Publishing, Cork.

Orla Kelly Publishing
27 Kilbrody
Mount Oval,
Rochestown
Cork,
Ireland

To Cathy, Ross, Ellie and Anna who have taught
me more about wellbeing than any book, podcast, or
programme ever could.

Reviews

'Tired of being tired?
Ready to move from Exhausted to Energised?
Ready to get back a life of greater joy, passion, focus and ease?
Your Wellbeing REVAMP is a powerful, practical guide for anyone ready to truly transform how they think, live and work.
Séamus masterfully blends science with soul, offering powerful daily habits that make a profound difference in how we feel, think and live.
This book doesn't just inform, it inspires, motivates, and equips you with the tools to thrive.
I highly recommend it to anyone serious about taking ownership of their wellbeing and living with greater clarity, energy, and purpose.'

— Gerry Hussey, Performance Psychologist & Founder of Soul Space

'Your Wellbeing Revamp is an evidence-led, refreshingly clear guide that makes the science of wellbeing practical and accessible to all. Séamus has struck the perfect balance of grounded research, written in a way that speaks to real, everyday life. A valuable tool for anyone looking to reset, recharge, and move forward with clarity.'

— **Dan Glynn, Mental Performance Coach, Monaghan GAA Senior Football Team**

'This book is so relevant, practical, and easy to engage with, making it a valuable resource for anyone looking to improve their wellbeing.'

— **Tony Óg Regan, Performance & Wellbeing Coach**

About the Author

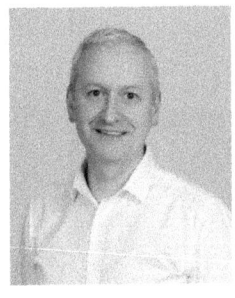

Séamus Ruane is a seasoned community pharmacist with a passion for promoting wellbeing through education and lifestyle change. Over the course of his career, he has witnessed the profound impact that lifestyle choices can have on health; both positively and negatively. Motivated to address the rising trend of lifestyle-related illnesses, Séamus founded iThrive to empower individuals and organisations to adopt practical, manageable steps towards long-lasting vitality and life satisfaction.

Séamus combines his professional expertise with an impressive portfolio of specialised training. He has studied stress management, yoga, and clinical hypnosis; holds a certificate in applied positive psychology from the Flourishing Center in New York; an internationally recognised leader in positive psychology training.

Through iThrive, Séamus offers a wide range of programmes designed to enhance wellbeing, including personal and corporate coaching through Your Wellbeing Toolkit, The iThrive Wellbeing Experience, The iThrive

Roadmap, and tailored workshops addressing building resilience and work-life balance. Each programme is thoughtfully designed to help participants reevaluate their approach to diet, exercise, stress, and success; areas where neglect is often normalised by society despite its detrimental impact on health.

Séamus's work has already left a lasting impression; he has received glowing feedback from participants, who describe his sessions as '*informative, engaging, and thought-provoking.*' He is committed to helping you invest in the most important asset of all; your wellbeing.

Who This Book Is For

Have you ever felt like you're running on empty; pushing forward, meeting deadlines, handling responsibilities, yet somehow never feeling truly *well*? You wake up tired, go through the motions, and wonder if this is just how life is supposed to be.

You're not alone.

In our modern world, the pressure to succeed, perform, and keep up is relentless. We tell ourselves we'll slow down *after* the next big project, *after* the kids are older, *after* we finally get that promotion, or *after* we reach some vague milestone that always seems just out of reach. But when does *after* ever really come?

For many high achievers, wellbeing feels like a luxury; something we'll get to once we've handled everything else. But here's the truth: Your wellbeing isn't a bonus; it's the foundation of everything. Without it, success feels empty, relationships suffer, and life loses its spark.

That's why this book exists.

I created *Your Wellbeing Revamp* because, as a community pharmacist and certified positive psychology practitioner, I've seen too many people: leaders, professionals, parents, business owners, people from all walks of life and backgrounds; pushing themselves to the brink, believing that stress and exhaustion are simply part of the price they have to pay to get through the daily grind and hustle. And I've learned that true success doesn't come from working harder, doing more, or sacrificing yourself. It comes from working smarter, being present, and aligning your energy with what truly matters.

This book introduces you to the REVAMP method; a simple yet powerful framework for reclaiming your wellbeing in a way that fits your real life. You'll discover how to:

- Strengthen your relationships to feel supported, connected, and valued
- Find deeper engagement in your work and daily activities
- Boost your vitality with sustainable habits that energise your mind and body
- Cultivate awareness to break free from stress cycles and make intentional choices
- Transform your mindset to build resilience, confidence, and emotional balance
- Rediscover your purpose to bring meaning and fulfilment into your daily life

This isn't another book telling you to '*just meditate more*' or '*wake up at five a.m. to be successful.*' It's a practical guide that acknowledges the reality of busy lives and provides strategies that are realistic, sustainable, and actually work.

Whether you're feeling overwhelmed and burned out or you simply want to elevate your wellbeing to thrive in all areas of life, this book will give you the tools to create lasting change; without guilt, without unrealistic expectations, and without having to overhaul your entire life overnight.

Your wellbeing revamp starts now. Are you ready?

Table of Contents

Introduction 1
    Take Your Wellbeing Temperature 5
    R – Relationships 9
    E – Engagement 10
    V – Vitality 11
    A – Achievement 12
    M – Meaning 12
    P – Positive Emotions 13
    Measure Your Wellbeing 14
    The Power of 1% Gains 19
    Story: The Coffee Cups 21

Chapter 1: Building Compassion and Kindness 23
    The Importance of Relationships for Wellbeing 23
    Practical Steps to Deepen Your Relationships 33
    Story: The Bed by the Window 36

Chapter 2: The Science of Mindfulness 39
    The Impact of Being Present in Your Daily Life 39
    Mind Full or Mindful? 45
    Choosing Calm in the Midst of Chaos 48
    Story: The Potato, the Egg, and the Coffee Beans 58

Chapter 3: The Joy of Exercise 61
Movement as a Key to Lifelong Happiness.......................... 61
9 Tips to Get Moving 74
Story: Sharpen Your Axe 78

Chapter 4: Discover and Apply Your Strengths........ 81
Discovering Strengths to Boost Wellbeing.......................... 81
List of Twenty-Four Strengths 85
Unlocking the Power of Strengths for Wellbeing 85
Signature Strengths 92
Using Strengths for Better Communication....................... 96
Story: The Teacher's Mistake 101

Chapter 5: The Search for Meaning 103
Coherence 105
Purpose.. 106
Significance 107
The Role of Values 108
Finding Meaning in Work 114
Story: The Three Stonecutters.. 115

Chapter 6: The Power of Breath............................. 119
The Mechanics Of Breathing 120
The Benefits Of Nasal Breathing...................................... 122
Sunrise Breaths.. 125
Balance Breaths 127
Sunset Breaths 128
Story: The Calm Archer 130

Chapter 7: Understanding Our Thoughts 133
Thinking Traps 134
Sentence Starters 141

  Catastrophising 142
  Story: The Glass of Water 146

Chapter 8: The Power of Positive Emotions 149
  Chosing Our Emotional State 154
  The Power of Gratitude 161
  Three Good Things 166
  Story: Happiness Is Within You 168

Chapter 9: Creating Change 171
  Knowledge vs Applied Knowledge....................171
  The Habit Loop..173
  Story: The Starfish Story 177

Bonus Chapter 179
  Key Takeaways 179
  Mindset Shifts 180
  Action Items...181

Free Gifts 183
Take the Next Step Towards Transforming Your Wellbeing 183
References 185

Introduction

Enjoy the little things in life because one day you'll look back and realise they were the big things.

—Kurt Vonnegut

I have always had a keen interest in health and lifestyle, which is probably why I studied to become a pharmacist. Topics that have long fascinated me include diet, exercise, meditation, stress management, emotions, and relationships and how these different factors weave together to determine the level of wellbeing we experience throughout our lives.

I'm not exactly sure where this interest stems from, but one event from my early career as a pharmacist struck a chord with me. It wasn't a dramatic bolt-of-lightning type event; in fact, it was quite the opposite; a normal, everyday, routine sequence of events.

I was working in my pharmacy in Galway when two guys, both of whom I knew, though neither knew the other, came into the pharmacy. Both were of a similar age, weight, and profile. Coincidentally, both had the same prescription for the same medication, same dose, same strength, identical in every way.

The medication in question was a statin used to lower blood cholesterol. The first guy came in; let's call him Frank; and he said, *'Séamus, can you get this prescription ready for me? I'll be back for it in five minutes.'* Off he went about his business, and I proceeded to prepare the prescription.

Five minutes later, true to his word, he returned to collect his medication. As he entered, the place immediately filled with that mouthwatering aroma of freshly battered fish and chips doused in salt and vinegar. You know that smell when the vinegar soaks into the paper bag? Irresistible! Now, remember, he was coming back to collect his prescription for cholesterol-lowering drugs, and under his arm he was carrying the equivalent of a brown paper bag full of cholesterol!

A couple of hours later, the second guy; let's call him Walter; presented with the same prescription. Walter was of a similar age, similar weight, and similar profile. *'Séamus, can you fill this prescription for me? But before you do, can I ask a couple of questions? Can you tell me a little bit about that medication? How does it work? Are there any supplements I should be taking? And what about my diet? What should I avoid, and what should I increase? Does exercise affect your cholesterol, and what about stress?'*

He was very interested and motivated to make changes and reduce his cholesterol levels. So we had a great chat about the various factors influencing cholesterol, and off he went with his medication.

It is what happened over the next six to twelve months that fascinated me and changed how I look at health, lifestyle, and daily choices; forever. Frank returned to the pharmacy once a month, and after a couple of months, his statin dose was increased. After another couple of months, aspirin was added to his prescription to keep his blood thin. After another few months of blood pressure medication came a diagnosis of type 2 diabetes, which meant he had to prick his finger a couple of times daily to measure his blood sugar level and take more medication to keep it within the desired range.

Compare this situation to Walter. He returned to the pharmacy once a month for about six months and then never set foot in the pharmacy again. His lifestyle interventions had corrected his cholesterol levels and sent him off on a completely different health trajectory.

That simple, everyday incident fascinated me and grabbed my attention. I wondered if lifestyle choices could have such a profound effect on cholesterol, would the same apply to other health conditions? I started to investigate and, of course, found that our daily habits and choices do have a profound effect on many health conditions. Extrapolating from that, I wondered if the same could be said for our happiness, our satisfaction with our lives, and our sense of wellbeing in general.

This is when I started investigating topics such as yoga, stress management, clinical hypnosis, and applied positive psychology. And no matter what I studied or investigated, the answer always seemed the same.

What we do on a daily basis, the choices we make, and the habits we instil in our lives are very real determinants of the level of happiness and wellbeing we experience throughout our lives. They really are the difference that makes the difference, as opposed to what we focus on; our achievements, our possessions, or our status in society.

Take Your Wellbeing Temperature

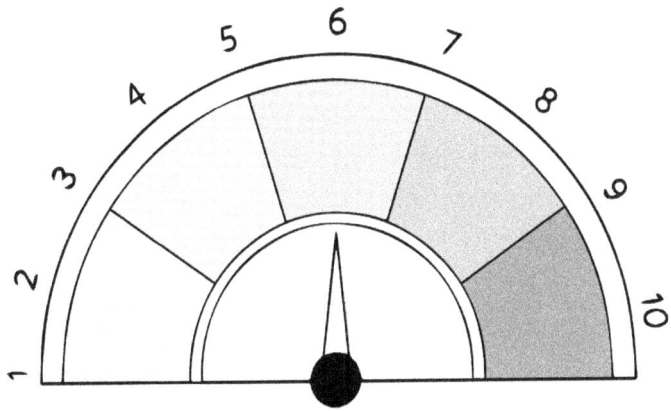

If you were to take a moment and assess your current state of wellbeing, where would it fall? On a simple scale from one to ten, with one representing feelings of stress, anxiety, and struggle, and ten reflecting a state of health, energy, happiness, and thriving in all areas of life, what number would you choose?

For many of us, the answer may reveal that there's always room for improvement. Wellbeing isn't something fixed or constant. It naturally ebbs and flows, influenced by the daily challenges and experiences we encounter. But what exactly is wellbeing, and how do we measure it? The term is used in a variety of contexts and means different things to different people. From wellbeing crystals to tarot cards in alternative stores, the concept can sometimes feel abstract. Yet, understanding wellbeing in a meaningful way is key to improving it in our own lives. I've also seen wellbeing referred to in articles in the *British Medical Journal* and *Journal of the American Medical Association*. It's easy to see how this can confuse people. How can one term be applicable to such a wide range of topics?

I suspect if you're reading this book, you have a keen interest in the concept and are probably committed to boosting your wellbeing. Still, if I were to ask you to define wellbeing, you might struggle to do so.

So I prefer to ask the following question: When it comes to your wellbeing, what is the number-one thing that you do that boosts it? This gives us an indication of what you feel your wellbeing is all about. In general, we find that our wellbeing is made up of various factors rather than a single factor alone.

Wellbeing is our ability to feel good and function effectively.
— Dr. Felicia Huppert

This is the definition of wellbeing I work with. I find it relatable, practical, clear, and simple. When it's defined this way, isn't it so obvious it's something we all want for ourselves, our friends, our families, and our loved ones? Sometimes wellbeing gets a bad rap as being a lightweight topic, but there's nothing fuzzy, flaky, or hippie-dippie about it for me. We're talking about something that's core to our experience as human beings.

I believe nothing in your life is more important than your wellbeing. Regardless of what you have, what you possess, or what you achieve, it all becomes utterly meaningless unless you can enjoy it and are able to function effectively.

Positive psychology is the scientific study of wellbeing. It is a relatively new science that has existed since 1998. Years of high-quality research since its inception have given us a wealth of data, tools, techniques, and interventions that have been validated and proven by science to have a positive influence on our level of wellbeing. Having trained in the health science field, I am confident in recommending these practices. We know if we incorporate the tools recommended into our daily lives, they will work!

Even with this knowledge, I still find there are impediments to people taking real action. When I ask someone why wellbeing isn't a higher priority in their lives, in general I get one of two responses. The first reason is so predictable. What do we all feel we don't have enough of? Time! *'I'm just too busy at the moment,'* *'We have a new baby,'* *'We're building a new house,'* *'Work is hectic at the moment,'* and *'When the kids get a bit older'* have been among the many reasons I hear.

People assume that it's going to take this enormous investment of time to look after their wellbeing and to change things. And because they see it as this big mountain to climb, they feel overwhelmed and paralysed and end up not taking any action. However, the science of wellbeing shows us that the consistent application of small daily habits is what actually boosts our wellbeing. Many of the habits we discuss in this book will take you less time than it takes you to brush your teeth daily. We're talking about just a couple of minutes a day.

The second response I get when I ask people why wellbeing isn't a greater priority is that they don't know where to start. *'I'd love to boost my wellbeing. I'm really interested, but I'm a bit confused; I just don't know where to start.'* People often ask for a road map, a format, or a model they can use. They want to have the confidence that if they invest resources such as their time, money, and energy into this, they will see positive results.

Positive psychology employs a model originally developed by Martin Seligman, widely regarded as the founding father of the scientific study of wellbeing. This framework has been further refined by other researchers over time, enhancing its relevance and adaptability.

The model I use identifies six areas of our lives that contribute to our overall sense of wellbeing. For ease of recollection, I like to use the acronym REVAMP, with each letter standing for a different area or pillar, as follows:

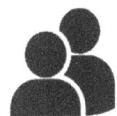 # R – Relationships

Research shows that the number-one thing you can do to boost your level of wellbeing is to increase the quality of your relationships. Evolution has hardwired us as human beings to connect with each other. Relationships include our connections with family, friends, neighbours, work colleagues; in fact, everyone we interact with daily.

It is so important that we never take our relationships for granted and that we constantly nurture and nourish them, because they are huge determinants of our level of wellbeing.

EXERCISE

Close your eyes for a moment and think of one of your life's highlights or high points so far. Now answer this question: Was that time or event in your life one that you spent on your own, or was it something you shared with someone else? For most people, it's an event or time they shared with someone. Relationships act as a multiplier in our lives, accentuating the good times.

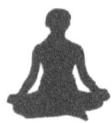 # E – Engagement

Engagement involves being fully present in your life. So, whatever activity you're partaking in, whether it's work, interacting with your family, or exercising, are you invested in the activity, fully present and aware, or are you just passing the time, ticking boxes?

Even though we can only exist in the present moment, our mind spends lots of time in the past and lots of time in the future. So, maybe as you read this book, you're thinking about what will happen later today, or what you'll have for lunch, or what you'll do this evening. Or are you thinking about what happened yesterday, last weekend, last week, last month, or last year? The more we're present and in the moment, the richer our life experience and the higher our levels of wellbeing.

A Harvard study on mindfulness highlighted a profound insight: *'a wandering mind is an unhappy mind.'*[1] This reinforces the importance of being present in the moment. When we focus deeply, we increase the chances of experiencing flow states; those instances of complete absorption in an activity. These moments not only enhance our engagement but also significantly boost our overall wellbeing.

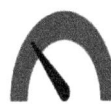 V – Vitality

Vitality is the energy to go about your daily life. Lots of things affect our vitality level, but there are three main ones: diet, movement, and sleep.

Diet

Our cells are constantly replaced, regenerated, and repaired. For these processes to occur, the body relies on raw materials, which are provided by the food we eat. Ideally, our food should come from sources as close to nature as possible.

Movement

We know that exercise leads to immediate changes in our physiology, body chemistry, and mood, but we also know that over the long term, the effects of exercise are enormously beneficial to both physical and mental health.

Sleep

Sleep is about much more than rest. When we sleep, our brains largely remain active. Lack of sleep is associated not only with poor mood but also with depression, obesity, and poor cardiovascular health.

 # A – Achievement

This involves setting, working towards, and achieving goals that are inherently important and motivating for you. People often think that achievement, possessions, and success are the routes to success, happiness, and wellbeing, and they focus all their efforts on these areas. As a result, their lives can often be about pursuing one goal after another, and when one is achieved, they move on to the next goal, and then the next goal, and so on.

It all becomes about doing more and more, but as is evident from the REVAMP model, achievement is only one area of six. Our lives need to be balanced, and we need to address all six pillars to lead a life of high wellbeing.

 # M – Meaning

Do you feel that your life has a clear sense of meaning and purpose, and are your daily actions aligned with it? Meaning doesn't have to be grand or monumental; it can be found in the small, meaningful actions of everyday life. Whether it's nurturing relationships as a father, mother, sibling, or friend, or using your unique skills to contribute positively to your community, these purposeful acts can profoundly enhance wellbeing. The more connected we are to a sense of purpose, the higher our overall sense of fulfilment and satisfaction in life.

 P – Positive Emotions

Positive emotions like excitement, enthusiasm, love, joy, awe, interest, and pride play a significant role in our wellbeing. The more we experience these emotions, the stronger our sense of happiness and fulfilment can become. But their importance goes beyond just feeling good. Positive emotions actively shape how our brain and nervous system function, influencing how we perceive and interpret the world around us.

Many people mistakenly believe they're stuck with the emotions they wake up with or experience throughout the day. For instance, starting the morning feeling grumpy might seem like something you just have to endure until it naturally fades. However, the truth is, we have the power to shift our emotional state with simple, effective strategies. Actions like using affirmations, listening to uplifting music, engaging in exercise, or reaching out to a friend can make a real difference. These tools are accessible, practical, and can help us feel better in the moment.

Now, this isn't about trying to be happy all the time; life's ups and downs are inevitable, and nobody is immune to them. However, with a bit of mindful effort, it's entirely possible to infuse more excitement, love, awe, and joy into your daily routine. Even small changes in how we approach our emotions can create a meaningful and lasting impact on our overall wellbeing. Why not take a moment today to explore one of these practices? You might be surprised at how much brighter things can feel.

To make this concept even more tangible, it can be helpful to use a structured, research-backed framework as a guide. This provides a clear roadmap to better understand and measure our wellbeing. At the start of this book, we used a simple one-to-ten scale to reflect on our overall sense of wellbeing. Now, with the REVAMP model, we have a tool that allows us to score ourselves across specific areas. This makes it easier to identify where we're already thriving and where there's room for growth, enabling us to focus our efforts more effectively.

Measure Your Wellbeing

Think about your experiences and feelings over the last week or month. How often has each of the following occurred? 0 = never, 5 = half the time, 10 = all the time

Pillar	Definition	Score
Relationship	I felt respected, appreciated and connected.	
Engagement	I was interested and deeply engaged in my activities.	
Vitality	Physically, I felt strong and healthy.	
Achievement	I made progress towards reaching my goals.	
Meaning	I felt my life had a sense of meaning and purpose.	
Positive Emotion	I felt positive and cheerful.	

It becomes evident to us, using this model, that our wellbeing is very much our own responsibility. The idea of going to a doctor or any health care provider and handing them the responsibility for our health and wellbeing belongs to a different era. Modern health care is based on an a treatment model focusing mainly on illness, sickness, and disease. Nobody walks into their doctor's surgery and says, *'Hello, Doctor, I'm feeling fantastic today, absolutely wonderful, brilliant in all respects, and I just thought I'd come in to let you know!'* That's not how it works, because medicine and health care are all about what's wrong, what's broken, what's diseased, and how we can fix it. You only engage with the health care system when there's something wrong or you are experiencing signs and symptoms of illness and disease.

Let's consider the patient's experience. When you feel perfectly healthy and symptom-free, you typically have no reason to engage with healthcare services. However, as soon as you start noticing signs or symptoms of illness, you may seek support from a healthcare professional; whether it's a doctor, nurse, psychologist, or another provider; depending on the nature of your concerns. They might diagnose the issue and outline a course of treatment. If the treatment is entirely successful; a major assumption; the best possible outcome healthcare can achieve is to bring you back to a state of neutrality. Neutrality means there is nothing wrong with you, and once you're no longer engaged with healthcare services, their role is considered complete. However, in positive psychology, we propose that a lack of illness does not necessarily equate to the best possible outcome. There is more to wellbeing than simply the absence of problems.

While healthcare is all about what's wrong, broken, and diseased, wellbeing is more concerned with what's good, what's working, what's strong, and how can I have more of that in my life.

What sets people who truly thrive and flourish apart from the rest? If we take a closer look at their habits, behaviours, and strategies, could we adopt their techniques to elevate our own lives and experience greater wellbeing?

Absolutely, we can. By learning and implementing these proven methods, we create a buffer that protects us from the signs and symptoms of illness or disease. Wellbeing should be at the core of your life, as it has the power to transform every aspect of how you live. The rewards of prioritising your wellbeing are extraordinary.

High levels of wellbeing aren't just about feeling good; they are directly linked to measurable improvements in your health. From a stronger immune system and better cardiovascular health to increased energy, reduced stress, and even less pain, the benefits are endless. And let's not forget, nurturing your wellbeing might just help you live a longer, more vibrant life. Remember, your wellbeing isn't a luxury or an afterthought; it's the foundation for a happier, healthier you.

When it comes to work, we are more productive and more engaged, get better customer service ratings, are more likely to be promoted, make better leaders, are more satisfied with our jobs, and are less likely to quit or burn out.

When it comes to our personal lives, we experience more fulfilling relationships and more positive emotions; we typically achieve more and have greater energy levels. There's no area that higher wellbeing doesn't affect. There is also a strong correlation between our wellbeing and our resilience. I like to think of this as putting money in the bank for the rainy day. When we have high levels of wellbeing, we are far better able to cope with the stresses and strains of work, and when challenges present in our lives, we are far better able to manage and to deal with them effectively.

We are all familiar with the saying, 'Knowledge is power.' However, I don't believe this to be entirely true. Knowledge on its own is simply interesting. How often have we read a book, watched a movie, downloaded an app, or listened to a podcast, only to do absolutely nothing with that information? Knowledge only becomes powerful when we choose to take action and apply it. That's when the real transformation begins. It's one thing to read this book from beginning to end, but it's entirely different to put its teachings into practice in your own life. Consider this analogy; knowing everything about fitness, including workout techniques, nutrition plans, and supplements, won't make a difference unless you put that knowledge to use. Only through consistent application will you start to see changes in strength, tone, and overall health. The key takeaway is this: while knowledge can spark our curiosity, it is applied knowledge that truly holds the power to create change.

The Power of 1% Gains

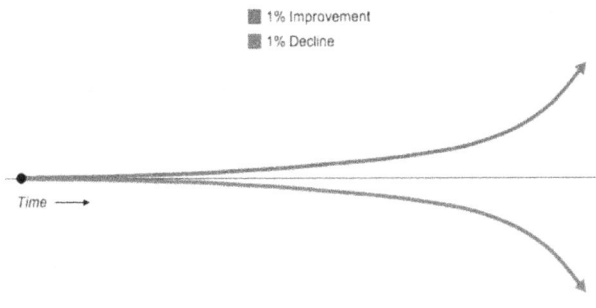

The Power of 1% Gains

Investing just a couple of minutes a day can significantly enhance your wellbeing. The principle of 1% gains proves that small, sustainable improvements bring remarkable results over time. You don't need drastic lifestyle changes or retreats to the Himalayas; the key lies in consistent, repeatable actions.

Minor actions may seem insignificant at first, but their power lies in repetition. A single attempt might yield no immediate effect, but repeated daily over weeks, months, or years, these small steps create a profound, lasting impact. It's like compound interest working in your favour. Conversely, minor errors in judgment, repeated over time, can lead to negative outcomes.

What will you do today to improve your wellbeing? Don't just read these ideas; take action. Start small. Consider one damaging habit you can quit. Is it excessive scrolling on social media? Evening snacking on the couch? Sacrificing sleep night after night? What simple activity could you begin? A walk, a swim, gardening, or catching up with friends? Identify one healthy habit you already practise. Commit to maintaining it. Is it staying hydrated, eating balanced meals, or regular exercise?

Research shows higher levels of wellbeing enhance relationships, work performance, and health. Wellbeing is far from being a fluffy, trivial topic; it's vital for thriving in life.

Many of us, however, neglect this in the rush of daily life. We wake up, jump onto the treadmill of routine, and rarely pause to reflect on what's truly important. Take a moment. Reflect. Choose one small, positive step today and see how it compounds over time.

Story: The Coffee Cups

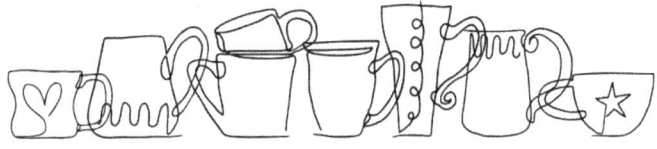

A group of college friends gathered at the home of their favourite college professor to celebrate his retirement. They hadn't seen each other in many years, and some had lost contact completely. Throughout the evening, they shared stories of where their lives had taken them; about their careers, families, and achievements. Before long, the conversation turned to the various challenges, stresses, and pressures they experienced.

As the evening progressed, the professor asked who would like a cup of coffee, and after taking the order, he went to the kitchen to prepare the required number with his wife.

A couple of minutes later, the professor and his wife emerged from the kitchen with two trays of steaming-hot coffee. The coffee was served in various cups: crystal cups, glass cups, ceramic cups. Some were shiny, some plain looking; some were ordinary, some were exquisite and expensive. After handing the coffee around, the professor noticed how all the nice cups were taken first and the ordinary ones were left to last.

The professor pointed this out to the college friends, saying, '*I notice you all wanted your coffee from the best cups, and this desire reflects the source of much of your dissatisfaction, problems, and stress in life. You see, the cup itself adds no quality to the coffee. When you think about it, you want the coffee, not the cup.*'

And so it is in life: Your life is the coffee, and your career, money, status, and position in society are the cups. The type of cup you have doesn't define or change your life quality, so don't let the cup drive you. Instead, focus on *enjoying* the coffee. Most people concentrate on the cup and fail to enjoy the coffee. Savour the coffee and not the cup, because no cup can compensate for bad coffee.

The happiest people in this world don't necessarily have the best of everything; they make the best of everything.

—Unknown author

CHAPTER 1

Building Compassion and Kindness

Tool: Kindness
Pillar: Relationships

You will be remembered more for your kindness than for any level of success you could possibly gain.

—Mandy Hale

The Importance of Relationships for Wellbeing

The first pillar in the REVAMP model of wellbeing is R, which stands for Relationships. The number-one thing we can do to boost the quality of our wellbeing is to improve the quality of our connection and our relationships with others. Our relationships include friends, family, work colleagues, neighbours, intimate partners, and indeed, anyone we interact with.

Chris Peterson, one of the founding fathers of positive psychology, was giving an interview to a journalist about the various aspects of wellbeing and positive psychology. The journalist, recognising that this was a vast field, asked Chris to briefly summarise the subject for him. Chris replied that he could summarise it in just three words: '*Other people matter.*' Such was the level of importance that he ascribed to relationships when it came to boosting our overall level of wellbeing.

Instinctively, we recognise the truth of that three-word summary. When someone is bereaved, for example, they often describe their life as being empty and pointless. Children who are brought up in institutions where they have no sense of belonging often appear withdrawn and frightened. And to shun someone or to exclude someone from your social circle is one of the most hurtful things you can do to another human being. At a deep level, we know that the bonds we form with other people are essential to our existence.

There are many phrases to reflect this undeniable fact. John Donne said, '*No man is an island.*' Aristotle called human beings '*the social animal,*' explaining that the one thing that distinguishes us from other species is the depth of our social entanglements and interactions.

Human beings are naturally wired to connect with others, and these connections have profound effects on our wellbeing. When we bond with others, our bodies release oxytocin, often referred to as the 'love hormone' or 'cuddle hormone.' This chemical is not only produced during moments like breastfeeding or intimate relationships but also when we experience something as simple as seeing a cute baby. The release of oxytocin has several positive effects, including reducing anxiety, enhancing focus, and improving the functioning of our cardiovascular, immune, and nervous systems.

From an evolutionary perspective, these social bonds have always been crucial for survival. Our early ancestors thrived in small, cooperative tribes where individuals relied on each other for tasks such as hunting, gathering, and childcare. Human infants, unlike the young of many other species, are born extremely dependent and require extensive care. This dependence necessitated strong, stable relationships within the tribe, enabling humans to pass on their genes and thrive as a species. Over time, this innate need for connection became deeply embedded in our DNA.

Today, reflecting on our own 'tribe' or support network can have significant benefits. Identifying and appreciating the people we depend on for friendship, support, and advice enhances our sense of connection. Simple, thoughtful gestures; like sharing a coffee, sending a note, or spending time together can nurture these relationships and reinforce their importance in our lives. Science backs this up. Relationships are not just beneficial; they are vital to our health and happiness. One striking piece of evidence comes from the Grant Study, the longest-running research project in psychology. Beginning in 1938, this study followed participants throughout their lives, analysing various factors such as marriage status, exercise habits, diet, and more. The findings were clear and profound. Warm relationships had the greatest impact on happiness and longevity. Dr. George Vaillant, one of the study's lead researchers, summed up this monumental study with just five words: *'Happiness is love. Full stop.'*[2]

On the flip side, loneliness and social isolation are deeply damaging; comparable to smoking cigarettes in terms of their impact on health. Chronic loneliness is associated with higher stress hormones, depression, weakened immune function, and increased mortality.[3] Shockingly, it poses a greater risk to health than either obesity or physical inactivity.[4]

The power of connection extends beyond personal relationships and into the workplace. Research reveals that positive interactions with colleagues significantly enhance job satisfaction and productivity. For leaders, creating a culture where meaningful connections are encouraged is vital; not just for the wellbeing of their teams but also for overall performance and cohesiveness.

Investing in relationships is therefore essential for a fulfilling life. Developing meaningful connections requires small yet intentional actions, a mindset of kindness, and a genuine focus on others. Whether it's through supportive gestures or simply making time for loved ones, these efforts enrich not just our social bonds but also our health and happiness. It's clear that prioritising connection is one of the most impactful ways to nurture our wellbeing and live a truly vibrant life.

It is said that kindness is the food that nurtures our relationships. When we perform acts of kindness for others, benefits accrue, not only to the person we are kind to but also to ourselves in terms of boosting our levels of wellbeing. This makes kindness quite unique. With most wellbeing tools, there is a lag time before any beneficial effects are felt; not so with kindness. If you happen to be in bad form and you want to shift that negative emotion instantaneously, the number-one thing you can do is something kind, caring, or compassionate towards someone else. There's no lag time; you get to feel good immediately.

Throughout the ages, every single religion known to humankind has promoted the idea of being kind to your fellow man. The Dalai Lama said, '*If you want others to be happy practice compassion. If you want to be happy practice compassion.*' There is an old Hindi saying '*True happiness consists in making other people happy.*' What I love about those two quotes is that both of them recognise that doing kind acts is good not only for the person we're being kind to but also for ourselves.

Is this just wishful thinking, or does science back this up? Interestingly, science offers compelling evidence for the benefits of kindness. If we attach electrodes to the brains of two individuals; one performing a kind act and the other receiving it; we can observe an incredible phenomenon. Pleasure centres in the receiver's brain light up, as expected, but remarkably, similar regions activate in the brain of the giver as well. This is because acts of kindness trigger the release of oxytocin or endorphins, our feel-good hormones. Together, these create what scientists call the '*helper's high*,' a sense of joy and fulfilment that demonstrates how good it feels to do good.

But the benefits of kindness don't stop there. Amazingly, kindness also has a ripple effect. When an observer witnesses an act of compassion, they too experience a release of feel-good chemicals, leading to that warm, fuzzy feeling we often get when we see something kind or heartwarming. Be it a selfless act on television or something witnessed in person, the power of kindness extends to all who encounter it. Simply put, kindness isn't just beneficial for the receiver; it's equally rewarding for the doer and even the onlooker. Science proves that kindness is a gift that keeps on giving. So why does kindness have such a powerful effect?

1. **Amplifying Gratitude Through Kindness**: Kindness opens our hearts to gratitude, helping us appreciate the blessings we have. When we actively seek opportunities to show kindness, we cultivate a heightened awareness of our own good fortune. By choosing to extend kindness to others, whether through our time, energy, or resources, we signal to our subconscious that life is abundant and we have enough to share. This simple yet profound act reinforces a mindset of peace and contentment.

2. **Escaping Negativity by Focusing Outward:** Kindness shifts our attention away from personal struggles, allowing us to break free from cycles of overthinking and negativity. Our natural tendency is to ruminate on problems, often leaving us stuck. However, when we turn our focus outward and seek ways to uplift others, we disrupt this pattern. The act of kindness creates a refreshing sense of purpose and reminds us that joy isn't just about fixing our own problems but also about making someone else's world a little brighter.

3. **Seeing Others Through a Lens of Compassion**: Kindness transforms the way we view others. It softens our judgement and fosters empathy. Imagine walking past someone who is struggling, like a homeless person or an addict. Instead of jumping to blame or judgement, kindness encourages us

to consider their humanity and recognise that no one deliberately chooses hardship. It changes our perspective from *'Why don't they fix their life?'* to *'How can I understand and help?'* This shift builds bridges of empathy, making the world a little kinder.

4. **Strengthening Bonds Through Cooperation**: Every act of kindness deepens our sense of connection and interdependence. Often, kindness is met with kindness in return, creating a cycle of mutual support. Reflect on all the people who have shaped your life; from family to teachers, friends, and mentors. When we extend kindness, it's a beautiful way of reciprocating the kindness we've received and strengthening the bonds within our communities.

5. **Boosting Self-Worth Through Kindness**: When we help others, we see ourselves in a new, empowering light. Kindness becomes a mirror, reflecting back our strengths, resourcefulness, and ability to make a difference. It builds confidence, optimism, and a sense of purpose. Helping someone through a challenge not only improves their situation but also reminds us that we are capable, impactful, and valuable.

6. **Discovering Meaning and Purpose**: Kindness infuses our lives with deeper meaning. As Leo Rosten wisely observed, *'The purpose of life is not to be happy but to be useful.'* The act of seeking out

opportunities for kindness is the living embodiment of usefulness. Each compassionate gesture we make contributes to something greater, giving our lives a sense of purpose that transcends day-to-day routines.

7. **Creating a Ripple Effect of Positivity**: Kindness is contagious. When we show kindness, it inspires gratitude in others, sparking a chain reaction. What starts as a single act can ripple outward, transforming relationships, families, workplaces, and even entire communities. By simply choosing to be kind, we can ignite a movement of positivity that spreads far beyond what we can imagine.

In my work, I often discuss wellbeing with organisations and companies, and one of the most common topics people bring up is the *'atmosphere'* in their workplace. What I find particularly intriguing is the idea of this atmosphere. Where does it go when the office is empty, or when employees leave for the day? Naturally, it doesn't linger in the physical workspace, because the atmosphere is something we create and carry with us. Each of us shapes and influences it through our actions, attitudes, and interactions.

Kindness is one of the simplest yet most powerful ways to transform this atmosphere, whether at work, at home, or in our communities. Imagine a workplace with two hundred employees, where each person commits to one act of kindness a day for five days. That's a staggering one thousand acts of kindness each week; one thousand little gestures of positivity that ripple through the organisation. The transformation to the atmosphere would be nothing short of remarkable.

Kindness doesn't just create a better atmosphere; it transforms relationships, fosters teamwork, and builds resilience. Organisations that cultivate a culture of kindness can experience stronger collaboration, reduced stress levels, and increased job satisfaction among employees.

Similarly, in families or social groups, even a simple act of kindness can dismantle tensions, build trust, and deepen connections.

The true beauty of kindness lies in the fact that it's a positive-sum game. Unlike many aspects of life such as competition in business or sport, where one person's gain often means another's loss; kindness benefits everyone involved. The giver and the receiver both gain, creating a cycle of positivity and growth. And the best part? It's unlimited. No matter how much kindness you give, there's always enough to go around, with the power to uplift not just individuals but entire communities.

Science underpins this understanding. Studies like the Framingham Heart Study conducted from 1983 to 2003 reveal the ripple effects of our emotions and behaviours. As part of this study, researchers examined nearly 5,000 people and collected a substantial amount of data on physical and mental health. One of the most remarkable findings is that having a good friend who reports themselves as being happy and living less than one mile away increases your chance of reporting yourself as happy by 25%.[5]

What this means is that a single act of kindness doesn't end with the giver or receiver; it spreads, creating clusters of positivity and wellbeing. This contagious nature of kindness means that the small, intentional actions we take each day can lead to exponential growth in happiness and connection within our circles. Imagine how much healthier, more productive, and harmonious our environments could become if we all chose to bring kindness into every interaction, big or small. The power of kindness, then, lies not just in what it achieves in the moment but in the widespread, lasting impact it leaves behind.

Practical Steps to Deepen Your Relationships

How do we go about practicing kindness and compassion and making it more visible and prominent in our lives? It is true that no act of kindness, no matter how small, is ever wasted. The important thing is just to show up. We don't have to do anything miraculous or offer profound words of wisdom or solve everyone's problems. Kindness consists of having an orientation towards other people and realising that just one kind word can change someone's entire day. Every time we interact with another human being, we have no idea what kinds of problems they have, what kinds of issues they face, what kinds of challenges they're trying to overcome. It all starts with a simple shift in attitude, a realisation that everyone has problems, stresses, and difficulties, even the person who on the surface may appear to have everything sorted and under control. And so the smallest thing we can do matters, whether that's spending an extra minute chatting with someone, stopping to ask someone how their day is going, a simple smile, or even just making eye contact. So we aren't really talking here about making an intervention or a grand gesture, just an orientation towards others and making time to connect.

In the workplace, those brief five-minute conversations in the morning chatting with colleagues about their weekend, their family, or their hobbies are far more valuable than they might seem. They provide an opportunity to connect on a personal level, helping us to build genuine relationships. The more we engage with others, the more we come to recognise our shared humanity. Beneath it all, we all carry similar hopes, ambitions, worries, and fears, and recognising this can build a greater sense of unity and understanding.

Relationships aren't only about those who play a significant part in our lives but extend to every person we interact with. A great way to boost connection is to express gratitude to those who often go unnoticed in our lives but imperceptibly make our days easier and more pleasant. It could be the person serving us a cup of coffee, at the checkout in the supermarket, or sharing the lift.

It's also helpful to spot strengths in others and tune down our negativity bias when it comes to our judgements of those we interact with. Often our default is to notice and focus on others' faults and failings. Imagine how transformative it could be if we chose to focus on the positive qualities; what is good, strong, and admirable about others. What a powerful shift this could make to our interactions.

I also love the idea of doing a five-minute favour every day for someone. Often our reason for not making the required changes to boost our wellbeing is that we feel we don't have the time, but which of us can't spare five minutes? Small favours could be as simple as introducing people to each other, sending a colleague an article or link to a topic of interest to them, sending a card or text to say you're thinking of someone because you know they're going through a difficult time, or simply picking up the phone for a chat; just a simple intervention. We're talking really simple but effective actions that over time make all the difference to the quality of your relationships. As the Dalai Lama has said, *'Be kind whenever possible. It is always possible.'*

Story: The Bed by the Window

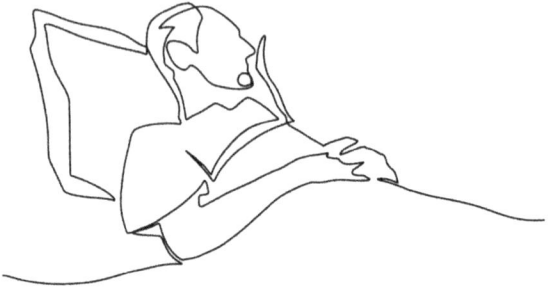

Two men, both seriously ill, were admitted to the same ward in the same hospital on the same day. One patient had a window bed, while the other one had a bed without access to a window or a view outside. The patient by the window was allowed to sit up for an hour every day to help drain the fluid from his lungs. The other patient had to spend the entire day, every day, flat on his back. The two men became friends and conversed about their families, friends, hobbies, and lives.

Every day when the patient by the window sat up, he described in great detail to his roommate all the beautiful things he could see outside the window. The patient in the other bed began to live for those one-hour periods where his world was brightened by all the activity and colour of the world outside.

The window overlooked a park with a lovely lake. The patient described how he could see ducks and swans swimming in the water, children playing excitedly in the playground, young couples walking arm in arm through flowers of every colour. In the distance was a magnificent view of a snowcapped mountain range. The patient on the other side of the room would close his eyes and imagine this picturesque scene.

Weeks later the patient was distraught when his friend by the window deteriorated rapidly and sadly passed away. He missed the way his roommate described the view from the window, and so after a few days, he asked the nurse to move him to the bed by the window.

The first afternoon in his new bed, he propped himself up on one elbow to look outside. To his surprise, the window faced a simple brick wall.

Confused, he wondered what had compelled his deceased roommate to describe such a beautiful and wonderful scene to him when, in reality, all that was there was a wall. He asked the nurse, who responded that the patient was in fact blind and couldn't even see the brick wall. She said, *'Perhaps he just wanted to make you happy.'*

In life, I think it's true that there is nothing more satisfying than seeing someone smile, and above all to know you are the reason behind that smile. Happiness is contagious, and the way it spreads from one human to another is by performing simple acts of kindness, caring, and compassion. Kindness boosts relationships, increases positive emotions, and gives meaning and purpose to our lives.

CHAPTER 2

The Science of Mindfulness

Tool: Mindfulness
Pillar: Engagement

> *Your calm mind is the ultimate weapon against your challenges.*
>
> —Bryant McGill

The Impact of Being Present in Your Daily Life

Next we're going to move on to the E in the REVAMP model, which stands for Engagement. Engagement is really just another word for present-moment awareness. We know when we boost our engagement, we boost our levels of wellbeing. Questions we need to ask here include *How present am I in my life? and How invested am I in what I'm doing?* This can apply to when you're working or when you're spending time with family or friends. Are you just going through the motions? Are you punching in the time but not really paying attention? While you're reading this book, is your mind wandering?

There is a phenomenon called *absence presence*, where we can be present physically but absent mentally. To what extent is that true in your life? And how can we boost our levels of engagement? A Harvard study on mindfulness concludes *'that a wandering mind is an unhappy mind.'* [1] When our brain is left to its own devices, it tends to focus on the problems, the mistakes, the threats, and all the difficulties in our lives, a phenomenon known as our *'negativity bias.'* This is what mindfulness helps us to do, to pull back from this tendency and create present-moment awareness.

The first step is to build up a level of self-awareness around our thoughts, our emotions, and our responses. The next step is to be agile with them. Can we make a shift and choose more helpful thoughts, emotions, and responses? Awareness always starts with slowing down.

In the modern-day world, I believe we suffer from what I term *social hypnosis*. Every day we get up in the morning and hop on the treadmill of life. We spend our hours, days, and weeks running and racing in an attempt to make everything bigger, faster, and stronger than it was last year. We expect more and more from ourselves and more and more from our lives. We have become so addicted to the treadmill we just assume it's normal, convincing ourselves *'that's just life.'* We live in a society where downtime, rest, and reflection are seen as being unproductive and lazy. But when we look at nature, we see that everything exists in cycles; night and day, summer and winter, the sun and moon, the tides coming in and going out. No system or organism exists in an *'always on'* state in the natural world. Busyness and action have to be followed with calmness and a sense of peace.

Mindfulness has become increasingly popular in the Western world over the last number of years. There are loads of articles, apps, podcasts, courses, and gurus out there instructing us on how to be more mindful and how we should incorporate meditation into our daily lives.

It is also implemented in a wide variety of settings, ranging from primary schools to prestigious institutions like Harvard University, and from the US military to the National Health Service in the UK. Over the past decade, it has gained significant traction and become much more mainstream. While this is undoubtedly positive, there are times when the buzz surrounding the *'next big thing'* can lead to some skepticism. People might dismiss it as merely a passing trend or a temporary craze, overshadowing its true value and potential.

However, mindfulness has a long and rich history that goes back thousands of years. Currently, it's being taken seriously by many multinationals and is the subject of much scientific research. It stands to reason that if something has lasted for thousands of years, there must be at least something to it.

Suggested benefits include:

- improved mood and focus, increased resilience, and decreased anxiety via boosting levels of serotonin and dopamine
- decreased stress levels, with those who meditate on a regular basis having lower cortisol levels.
- greater self-control and emotional intelligence
- improved connections with others (one type of meditation, called *loving-kindness meditation*, in which we repeat a mantra along the lines of '*May you be well, may you be happy, may you live in peace*,' results in the release of oxytocin.
- improved sleep
- diminished pain
- improved digestion
- greater heart health and blood pressure reduction
- boosted immune response

Obviously, these are hugely significant benefits. Many are mediated through engaging the parasympathetic nervous system, the part of our autonomic nervous system responsible for rest, rejuvenation, and repair in our body.

Exercise

I invite you to close your eyes for a moment, perhaps for about one minute, and turn your attention inward. Simply observe your thoughts as they arise and pass. Resist the urge to judge or control them; instead, approach them with curiosity and openness, noticing their flow without attachment.

And when you are ready, open your eyes. What did you notice about your thoughts? Most people observe that their thoughts are quite chaotic and seem to flit from one thing to something completely unrelated, never really settling on anything. The Buddha compared what's going on in our brains to a troupe of drunken monkeys, swinging from one branch to another, apparently completely out of control. When we consider what's actually occurring in our brains from a structural and biochemical point of view, this should come as no great surprise to us.

The human brain is an extremely complex organ. Scientists estimate that there are approximately one hundred billion neurons in your brain. A neuron is just a nerve cell that has a structure similar to a tree, with a trunk, branches, and roots. Neurons are arranged head to toe, with the branches of one tree being entangled with the roots of another. Each neuron is connected to multiple other neurons. It's estimated that there's one quadrillion connections in your brain, which is one thousand million, million connections, a number that is unfathomable to our limited minds. If you were to stretch out your brain cells end to end, they would cover a distance of roughly 1,000 kilometres. It's estimated that every single second, one hundred thousand chemical reactions occur in your brain. So we're talking about a degree of complexity that we can't even begin to comprehend.

It's said that when you consider the number of neurons in your brain, all the connections between neurons, and the fact that each connection can be turned on or off, there are more possible permutations and combinations than there are atoms in the entire universe! With this in mind, it can't come as a huge surprise that what's going on in there is quite chaotic. Indeed, that's what we found in the exercise when we closed our eyes and observed our thoughts for just one minute. So where does mindfulness fit into all of this?

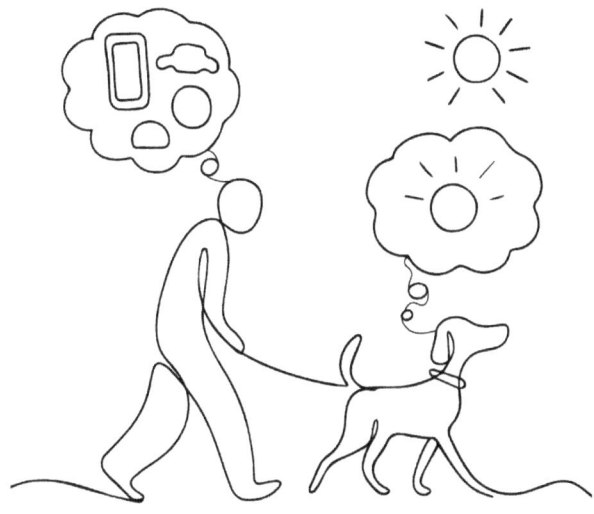

Mind Full or Mindful?

The cartoon above sums up things really nicely. In it, a human being is bringing their dog for a walk in the park. Both of them are having completely different experiences. The human's mind is full, lost in thoughts and concerns. They're not really taking in their current environment but preoccupied by concerns about work, traffic, finances, and relationship issues. Compare this to the dog. The dog is walking in the park, enjoying the brightness and heat from the sun with no distracting thoughts on their mind. So the human's mind is full while the dog is mindful. The dog is having a much richer experience than the human. In our lives, we spend most of our time not being truly present. And as a result, we miss the richness of our lives. We're there physically, but we're not there mentally. Mindfulness is simply how we go about bringing that present-moment awareness back to our lives. Eventhough we can only experience the world in the present moment, we spend lots of time thinking about the past, ruminating on something that happened five minutes ago or yesterday or last week or last year. Our minds also spend lots of time in the future. *What will I do after I finish reading this book? What's going to happen tomorrow? Next week? Next month? Next year? What happens if I get sick? What happens if I lose my job?* Mindfulness allows us to extend the length of time we spend in the present moment. And the more present we are in our everyday moments, the richer the experience we have of those moments and the more engaged we are with others and with life. Positive psychology shows us that the more engaged we are in our lives, the higher the level of wellbeing we will experience.

So what exactly is mindfulness? There are many misconceptions, so let's start off by saying what it isn't.

Mindfulness has nothing to do with being '*zoned out.*' It's not about being the most annoyingly positive person in the room! It's no longer considered alternative, and its application has become widespread all over the world. It's not religious, even though it has its origins in ancient Eastern religions. It's not really about relaxation, but sometimes relaxation is a side effect. It doesn't remove our sharpness. In fact, it does the exact opposite, because when we are mindful, we are so tuned in to what's happening in the present moment that it actually increases our sharpness and improves our focus. Mindfulness doesn't necessarily have to be time-consuming. You don't have to practice mindfulness for hours a day to see benefits.

If that's what mindfulness isn't, then what exactly is it? Jon Kabat-Zinn, a professor of medicine at the University of Massachusetts, is the person credited with bringing mindfulness to the Western world. He wanted to see whether, if he taught mindfulness to his patients, they would improve physically and mentally. He removed all religious connotations from mindfulness. His eight-week Mindfulness-Based Stress Reduction course is seen as the gold standard for learning mindfulness and is available worldwide.

He defines mindfulness as '*keeping our attention on our experience, from moment to moment, in an open and non-judgmental way.*' Firstly, we focus our attention on our experience. We experience the world through our five senses; what we see, smell, taste, touch, and hear. We can also pay attention to our breath. When we do so, we bring ourselves into the present moment. We do that on a moment-to-moment basis, which means we're focusing on, for example, this breath, then this breath, then this inhalation, this pause, and this exhalation. We do this in an open and non-judgemental way, meaning we don't assess whether the experiences are pleasant or unpleasant, boring or exciting. When we lose our focus (which we surely will) and get lost in thought, we don't give up, we don't criticise. We simply notice, and when we do, we bring our attention back to our breath.

Choosing Calm in the Midst of Chaos

Dan Harris was an anchor at ABC News and presented weekend editions of *Good Morning America*. He wrote a book and developed an app called 10% Happier. I really like the way he distils mindfulness down to its simplest form. He says that meditation is just '*noticing what's happening in your head at any given moment without getting carried away by it.*' Dan Harris led a high-powered, high-stress, busy, unbalanced lifestyle. One day live on TV, in front of tens of millions of people, he had a panic attack. He was really sceptical of complementary and alternative therapies but tried everything to help relieve him of his anxiety. The only thing he found to be of benefit was mindfulness. He now dedicates his time to convincing fellow sceptics to simply give it a go.

There are multiple books, apps, courses, and gurus explaining the details of mindfulness, but Dan Harris sums it up in three simple steps.

1. Sit comfortably with your back straight.

2. Focus your attention on your breath coming in and going out.
3. Bring your attention back to your breath. You don't have to clear your mind. Getting lost and coming back is the whole game.

For me, the part that most people miss is *'getting lost and coming back is the whole game.'* For many, this is the stumbling block, and people often say to me when I suggest introducing mindfulness into their daily routine, *'Séamus, I just can't meditate. I keep getting distracted. My mind keeps wandering.'* It's really important to understand that wandering is the nature of the mind. So whether you've been meditating for the last five days, five weeks, five years, or indeed fifty years, your mind is always going to wander. That's the nature of your mind. Your only job when you're practicing meditation or mindfulness is to bring your attention back to your breathing whenever you notice that it has wandered.

Saying you can't meditate because your mind keeps wandering is like saying that you went to the gym, lifted a weight, put it down again, and that it didn't work because your muscle is the same size! When you go to the gym and you lift repeatedly, you're exercising and building your muscle. Likewise, when we practice mindfulness and our mind drifts, when we bring our attention back to our breathing, it's like flexing our muscle of attention, or our awareness muscle. So if your mind keeps wandering and you keep bringing it back, you are practicing absolutely perfectly.

So why should we be bothered? Why should we actually care and put in the effort? There is growing evidence that our twenty-four-hours-a-day/seven-days-a-week chaotic, stressful lives, which have become the norm in the modern world, are doing us immense harm. We know that stress is a recognised cause and precursor to many different illnesses. We also know that our health and wellbeing can be significantly improved by taking the time to simply slow down.

We live in immensely challenging times. Humankind has been in existence on the planet for two hundred thousand years, but over the last ten to fifteen years, we have seen enormous lifestyle changes, mainly as a result of emerging technologies. Many people refer to the present age not as the age of technology but as the age of distraction.

For many, the idea of working nine a.m. to five p.m. Monday to Friday is a thing of the past. We have a blurring of the lines between our working lives and our leisure time. We exist in a constant flow of information. Our conditions are changing rapidly and there is less support for our basic human needs, such as sleep, rest, physical activity, and a sense of belonging. Many of the modifications that have occurred in our lifestyles are subtle, and when we live through them, we don't tend to notice them. So here's a little trip down memory lane for you.

Who remembers the television test signal? Imagine that a couple of decades ago, television used to close for the evening! When I talk to younger generations about this, they scarcely believe that at eleven p.m., the national anthem would play and the television would go black until the following morning. It sounds so archaic now when we think of on-demand streaming, always-on internet, twenty-four/seven news, social media, Instagram, Facebook, and TikTok, all accessible every single moment of every single day.

Who remembers a home phone or a landline, as we used to call them? A phone connected to an exchange via wires usually located on a table in the hall of almost every home throughout the country. The phone had a little bell, and if it rang and you were within earshot, you answered it, and if you weren't, the person on the other end didn't get through. There was no mechanism for leaving a message that they were trying to reach you; they would just try again later. Now, I realise that modern-day communication and technology is miraculous and comes with enormous benefits. But I also think we should be under no illusion that those advantages come at a price to us, and we pay that price by being constantly available, always on.

In my hometown, in my youth, shops used to close on Sundays and for a half day on Thursdays. Nine a.m. to six p.m. were the normal open hours. This gave a beginning, middle, and end to the day and to the week. I distinctly remember the car park in our local shopping centre being completely empty on Sundays except for a few learner drivers practicing to drive, and now Sundays are one of the busiest shopping days of the week. Now, one day, one week just blurs into the next. I believe that in today's society, it is so easy to become addicted to being busy.

Every morning, we hop onto the treadmill of life, and the treadmill is the default. When we're not busy, we think there's something wrong with us. Life has become all about progress, goals, and achievement. People constantly feel the need to strive; to have something, to be someone, to get something. In my own experience, I have found that introducing an element of calm, peace, and ease has been an absolute game changer. However, this goes somewhat against the grain of our society, which may see these states as unproductive, a waste of time, and even lazy.

Positive psychology suggests that the exact opposite is true, and that prioritising calm, peace, and ease actually makes us more productive. How could this be true, as it seems counterintuitive?

Our autonomic nervous system is that part of our nervous system responsible for processes in our body that happen automatically, that are not under our conscious control. For example, it's responsible for ensuring our heart is beating at the perfect rate, pumping oxygen to every single cell in our body. It ensures our blood vessels are at the exact right tension, such that if we were to stand up immediately, the tension would adjust to make sure blood continues to flow to our head, preventing us from collapsing in a heap. It ensures stomach enzymes and acid are being produced to digest our food. It regulates our hormones so that every single process in our body is happening perfectly.

There are two parts to the autonomic system, namely, the sympathetic nervous system and the parasympathetic nervous system. The sympathetic nervous system is responsible for our stress response, also known as our fight-or-flight response. It's active when we are stressed, anxious, busy, or we're on the treadmill of life. We can compare it to an accelerator in a car. The parasympathetic nervous system has an opposing effect and is all about rest, repair, and rejuvenation. It's active when we experience a sense of calm, peace, and ease. We can compare it to the brakes in a car.

Modern life is all accelerator and no brake. We have been hypnotised into thinking that life is all about progress, goals, achievements, striving for bigger, faster, and stronger. As a result, our bodies are completely out of balance. Over the long term, being out of balance can show up as sickness and ill health. We need to make sure we rebalance ourselves. We can't be all accelerator and no brake.

The largest nerve in the parasympathetic nervous system is called the vagus nerve. The vagus nerve has lots of innervations in the area of your abdomen. People who meditate regularly stimulate their parasympathetic nervous system and have high vagal tone. High vagal tone is associated with emotional resilience, less inflammation in the body, and a decreased incidence of heart attack.

The greatest gift that mindfulness offers us is the ability to extend the gap between stimulus and response. We think we feel the way we do because of circumstances that happen to us. For example, *'the traffic is heavy, so I'm getting anxious; work is busy, so I'm getting stressed; someone says something I don't like, so I'm getting angry.'* We think our emotion is caused by the circumstance or event and collapse the event and our reaction. In reality, there is a gap between the two, and mindfulness allows us to extend, or open up, that gap, allowing us to choose a response rather than simply reacting.

And so the traffic being heavy doesn't necessarily mean I have to get anxious; work being busy doesn't necessarily mean I have to get stressed; someone saying something I don't like doesn't necessarily mean I have to get angry. When we are mindful, we can create this space, allowing us to become more aware, which in turn allows us to respond rather than react. This ability to choose our reaction is essentially a large determinant of our emotional intelligence. For me, that's the greatest gift that mindfulness or meditation gives. The Buddha probably says it a little better than I can: *'In life, we cannot always control the first arrow. However, the second arrow is our reaction to the first. And with this second arrow comes the possibility of choice.'*

In practical terms, this translates as follows: You're extremely busy at work. Automatically, you might begin to experience a degree of stress or anxiety. When you're living mindfully, you're aware of that stress or anxiety as it happens. You are tuned in to how it feels in your body and in your physiology. Because you are mindful, you can then decide to be aware of the stress and anxiety but not to follow it, to choose a different, more helpful response. This alternative response is the *'second arrow,'* and you get to choose what this is. So you have the option to either follow your stress and anxiety and to maintain and perpetuate it for the next hour, or the next five hours, or the next five days, or you can just be that stressed person in the office. Alternatively, you can decide *I'm going to do something different. I am in charge of my thoughts, my emotions, and my reactions, and I choose calm, peace, and ease.* That to me is the greatest gift of meditation and mindfulness.

Exercise

Three Minute Guided Meditation

Find a comfortable position either sitting or lying down. Let your hands rest gently in your lap or by your sides.

Minute 1 – Grounding
Take a deep breath in through your nose….and slowly exhale through your mouth.
Again, breathe in deeply… and breathe out completely.
Let your eyes close gently if they haven't already.
Feel the ground beneath you, supporting you fully.
Notice the weight of your body and allow yourself to settle.

Minute 2 – Breathing
Now, bring your attention back to your breath.
There's no need to change it in any way, just notice it.
Feel the air moving in as you inhale, and out as you exhale.
If your mind starts to wander, gently return your focus to your breath without judgement or criticism.

Inhale...
Exhale...
Each breath is a chance to relax a little more.

Minute 3 – Presence
Now bring your attention to your body.
Notice any sensations; warmth, coolness, stillness.
Let your shoulders drop, and your jaw soften.
Let go of any tension you're holding throughout your body..

Take a moment to simply be, not needing to do anything, just to be here, now.

When you're ready, slowly begin to wiggle your fingers and toes.
Take one final deep breath in, and exhale gently.
When it feels right, open your eyes.

You've just taken a few moments to pause and reset. Remember to carry this calm with you into the rest of your day.

Story: The Potato, the Egg, and the Coffee Beans

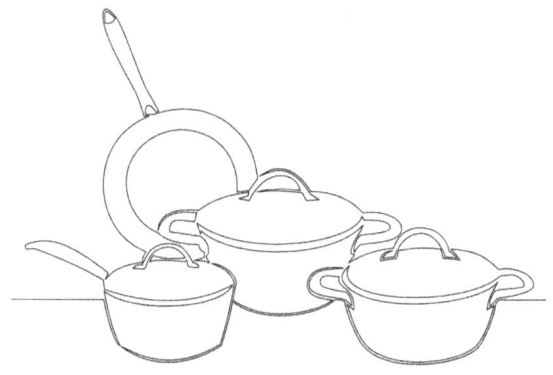

In a remote village lived a father, a mother, and their daughter.

The girl experienced many difficulties, misfortunes, and stresses throughout her life. One day she felt very depressed and overwhelmed about the extent of her stresses.

In the evening when her father, who worked as a chef in a local restaurant, came home, he sensed her low mood and despondency.

'*What's wrong, my dear?*' he asked gently.

'*My life has become so miserable, and I don't know what to do,*' she replied. '*I'm tired of fighting and struggling with my problems all the time.*'

Her father brought her to the kitchen and filled three small pots with water, then placed them on the cooker.

When they began to boil, he placed a potato in one, an egg in the second, and ground coffee beans in the third. After about twenty minutes he turned off the cooker, removed the potato and egg from their pots, and ladled the coffee from the third.

'*What do you see?*' he asked his daughter.

'*Potatoes, eggs, and coffee,*' she replied in exasperation.

'*Touch the potato and notice how it has softened,*' he said. '*Now take the egg and break it.*' After pulling off the shell, she observed the hard-boiled egg. '*Finally, sip the coffee,*' he said. Its rich aroma brought a smile to her face.

Her father explained, '*The potato, the egg, and the coffee beans have each faced the same adversity: the boiling water. However, each one of them has reacted differently. The potato went in strong, hard, and unrelenting, but in boiling water, it became soft and weak. The egg was fragile, with a thin outer shell, but inside, the egg became hard. However, the coffee beans were unique. They changed the water and created something new, something better.*'

'*Which are you?*' he asked her. '*When challenges knock on your door, how do you respond, and how can you respond in a more empowering way? Life is 10% what happens to you and 90% how you react to it.*'

Ultimately, it's not what happens to you that matters. What really determines what you become is your response to your stresses and challenges. Be mindful and aware of how you engage with and respond to everyday moments like these.

CHAPTER 3

The Joy of Exercise

Tool: Physical Exercise
Pillar: Vitality

Life has no remote . . . get up and change it yourself.

—Mark A. Cooper

Movement as a Key to Lifelong Happiness

The V in the REVAMP model stands for Vitality. Vitality is simply the energy to go about our daily business. It's what most people think about when I bring up the topic of addressing our wellbeing. There is a long list of factors that affect our vitality; a hierarchy of sorts. Three items occupy the top of that hierarchy: nutrition, sleep, and movement.

When it comes to nutrition, we know our cells are constantly dying off and new ones are constantly being created. Those new cells require a raw material, and this is provided by the foods we consume. So it's really important that the food we eat is as close to nature as possible; our bodies themselves are of nature. Essentially, this means that the less processed foods in our diet, the better.

The next important factor that influences our vitality is sleep. Sleep is about a lot more than just downtime, and when we sleep, our brains largely remain active. Sleep affects not just our brains but is also important for our immune system and our cardiovascular system. Lack of sleep can also have a significant effect on our mood.

Finally, movement and physical exercise have a profound effect on our overall vitality.

So much has been written about the various beneficial effects of exercise on our physical and mental health, and I have no intention of spending this chapter telling you what you already know: Moving your body is really good for you! Instead, I like to focus on some of the lesser-known and not-as-obvious benefits of physical exercise, so that when you become aware of the multitude of benefits associated with movement, you come to realise that it's impossible to have a wellbeing strategy that doesn't include physical movement.

No doubt we are all familiar with the long-term benefits of moving our body, but we also experience many immediate benefits. I am sure you are familiar with this scenario: You wake up in the morning tired, groggy, and lazy. You manage to convince yourself to go for a walk, run, cycle, or swim, and when you finish, you feel completely transformed. Vibrant, energetic, positive. I often think the person who goes for the run and the person who returns are almost two different people! Exercise transforms your attitude, outlook, and energy. Movement is a fantastic way to manipulate our body chemistry, change the expression of our nervous system, and manipulate our mood.

Remarkably, research shows that people who move their body on a regular basis are happier, more satisfied with their lives, have a stronger sense of purpose, experience more gratitude and more love, are more connected to their communities, and experience less loneliness and depression. These benefits occur throughout our lifespan, irrespective of our socioeconomic group or our culture. Most interestingly, these benefits aren't linked to our level of fitness but to the act of moving our body.

Movement, physical activity, exercise is like hitting the jackpot or winning the lottery for our body. Movement influences brain chemicals that give us energy, reduce worry, and help us to connect and bond with other people. It makes us more receptive to joy, increases our social connection, and reduces inflammation in our brain so we're less likely to experience depression, anxiety, or loneliness. These effects are embedded into our very physiology. When we exercise, our muscles secrete hormones that scientists call hope molecules, meaning that exercise actually makes us more optimistic and makes our brains more resilient to stress.

The entire setup of our body, our entire physiology, is engineered to reward us for moving. The obvious question to ask is why this is the case. The initial first guess people respond with is because movement has enormous health benefits. However, although true this doesn't take into account how movement has helped us to survive as a species. Throughout our evolution, we see that our bodies have been hardwired to take pleasure in any activities, experiences, or states that helped us survive as a species. For example, we take pleasure in eating, sleeping, teamwork, kindness, and compassion. Many scientists believe the reason we are rewarded when we exert ourselves is that movement is how we engage with life. It is suggested that the entire purpose of the human brain is to produce movement in our body, because that is the only way we can interact with the world.

As well as being rewarded chemically when we exert ourselves, we can also see that our bodies are literally designed to move. In what has to be the most amusing title of any academic paper, '*Why Is the Human Gluteus So Maximus?*' or, in layperson's terms, '*Why are our bums so big?*' David Lieberman, an anthropologist from Arizona,[6] outlines how the specific design of our body makes it obvious that we have evolved to move. He outlines how our gluteal muscles are large, our Achilles' tendons are long, and we have a large proportion of slow-twitch fibres in our muscles, all signs pointing towards the design of a body made to move. We even have a ligament called the nuchal ligament at the base of our skull that prevents our head from bobbing around when we run. This ligament is also found in wolves and horses, animals who are also designed to run.

Next, we must consider the motivation to move, because in the past, the human experience was all about preserving precious calories and energy. When resources were scarce and the source of our next meal uncertain, preservation of energy was an important factor to consider. This is why the runner's '*high*' exists, a reward for moving and persisting. It consists of the release into our body of endorphins, which are pain-reducing chemicals, and endocannabinoids, which result in the experience of increased pleasure and a desire to connect. Although some athletes describe the runner's high as a somewhat spiritual experience, I have also heard it described as being similar to downing two Red Bulls and vodka, swallowing three ibuprofen tablets, and finding a €1,000 lotto ticket in your pocket!

Interestingly, a slow walk or a short, intense bout of exercise doesn't trigger the runner's high. It requires a degree of persistent movement, such as jogging at an intensity similar to what our ancestors would have used for hunting. The runner's high is also triggered if we go hiking, swimming, cycling, or dancing, and the key to unlocking it is activity that is sustained for twenty minutes or more. This means it is probably more accurate to call this effect the persistence high rather than the runner's high, as it was designed to reward our hunter-gatherer ancestors to keep them hunting and keep them gathering.

A notable element of the runner's high is that as well as producing a feel-good element, it also promotes a sense of oneness and connection to others. The reason for this is thought to be that it encouraged our ancestors to share the spoils of the hunt with others in the group. This effect is produced by endocannabinoids, which make it more pleasurable for us to be around others, reduce social anxiety, and help us forge strong interpersonal attachments. Endocannabinoids can be called our *'Don't Worry, Be Happy'* chemicals. They regulate our stress hormones; dampen the activation of our amygdala, the fear-based part of our brain; and make us more content, mellow, and optimistic. In one study, when a substance called CCK-4 is injected into people, it precipitates a sense of panic and anxiety. If the subjects are allowed to exercise for thirty minutes prior to receiving the injection, it has an effect similar to taking a Valium tablet. Essentially, this suggests that moving our body can counteract anxiety that has been injected into our system. This often reminds me of how Wim Hof, the Iceman, often describes the transformative effects of breathing as *'getting high on your own supply.'* I think we can steal that quote to describe the effects of movement and exercise on our biochemistry.

In summary, when we move, an entire pharmacy of beneficial biochemicals and hormones are released into our system. Physiologically, our bodies are designed to move, and it is impossible to have a wellbeing plan that doesn't include movement and exercise. We cannot outrun our biology.

Now that we know all these amazing effects that moving produces in our physiology, how can we use movement as a tool to improve our wellbeing and not just see it as another item on our to-do list? How can we frame movement as a tool to help us feel better physically and mentally, to reduce stress, and to improve our vitality? Exercise is known as a keystone habit. This is simply a habit that leads to the development of multiple other good habits in our lives, similar to a domino effect. We know that people who exercise on a regular basis are more likely to have a healthy diet, more likely to be within the recommended weight range, more likely to be hydrated, and less likely to smoke. When we exercise, we see, firsthand, that our behaviour matters, leading us to make better choices.

When examining our ancestors' relationship to movement, it is clear that they never had to put on their running gear and say, *'See you later, I'm heading off for a run; I'll be back in about an hour!'* That wasn't the way it worked for them; moving their bodies was just an integral part of their lives. They were nomads and hunter-gatherers who were constantly on the move. We still exist in those prehistoric bodies, but do so in a very, very different world. The modern world is hyperfocused on convenience: How can we set up our environment to ensure we can minimise our movement? We have computers, cars, and washing machines that have completely changed how we work, how we commute, how we clean. Our lives have become increasingly more sedentary.

Thinking back one or two generations, our parents and grandparents tended to walk or cycle to school and went to the well for water. Most people were engaged in physically demanding labour. In today's world, technology has removed the need for movement so that now we can do the shopping, go to the bank, and order our clothes with a few keystrokes or the swipe of a phone. This remarkable increase in convenience and technology in our lives has also mirrored significant increases in lifestyle related diseases such as obesity and diabetes. Many health experts believe that we are facing a modern-day epidemic where physical inactivity in our lives now affects more people than smoking.

In our ultimate quest for convenience in the modern world, we have engineered physical activity out of our daily routines. Because of this, we've got to find ways to re-engineer it back in. In this context, it's useful to ask ourselves what our own relationship to exercise is. Do we exercise because we feel we have to, because we feel we should, or do we exercise because we just love it? Is there any particular exercise that we really enjoy?

When we consider the multitude of benefits of exercise, what immediately becomes obvious is how exercise boosts our physical resilience. Exercise places demands on various body systems and organs, and these systems and organs respond by becoming stronger and more efficient. What initially comes to mind in this regard are the significant cardiovascular benefits. When we exercise, we put more pressure on our heart, and our heart responds by becoming stronger. Physical movement puts increased pressure on our lungs, resulting in increased efficiency of our breathing.

Weight-bearing exercise causes microscopic tears in our bones, and our amazing body responds by repairing those tears, producing stronger and denser bones. In fact, the number-one recommendation for people who are at risk of osteoporosis is weight-bearing exercise.

Exercise also increases the plasticity of our blood vessels. When we exercise, our muscles have an increased requirement for oxygen, which is supplied by our blood vessels. As a consequence, exercise results in the formation of new blood vessels to cope with the increased requirement. The new blood vessels that are formed are more pliable and supple, and many health experts use the quality of our blood vessels as an indicator of our overall level of health.

Exercise also has a positive effect on the functioning of our immune system. While exercising, the change in our breathing pattern expels microbes that would otherwise stagnate in our lungs. Exercise also increases the production of antibodies and increases the production of white blood cells. Finally, the increase in body temperature associated with exercise makes our bodies less hospitable to bacteria and viruses.

Even though exercise involves the expenditure of energy, it also makes us more efficient at producing and storing energy. We can all relate to this effect; you're tired, lethargic, and unmotivated, yet you manage to go for a walk, a run, or a cycle. Paradoxically, even though you have used energy while moving, when you return, you're buzzing with energy, ready to take on the day. This is because exercise has a positive effect on your mitochondria. Mitochondria are called the energy powerhouses of our cells. Exercise can be shown to increase the number of mitochondria in your muscle cells, and this is thought to be how it results in greater muscle strength and endurance.

Also, surprisingly, even though we often think of lactic acid as a bad thing and associate it with muscle soreness that can be experienced after exertion, lactic acid actually travels to our brain and changes our neurochemistry, resulting in reduced anxiety and protection against depression.

All of these remarkable adaptive features of our body are great examples of the physical resilience of the human body. In essence, we put extra stress and pressure on our body, and our incredible body bounces back and responds to all the challenges by becoming more efficient, stronger, and healthier. And those are just the physical benefits. Just as impressive are the mental health benefits.

Exercise increases mitochondria not only in our muscle cells but also in our brain cells. This makes our brain cells more effective and efficient. Exercise is a valid component in the treatment or prevention of different mental health issues. We all know that exercise is beneficial for depression and has a positive effect when it comes to stress reduction.

Exercise results in the formation of new connections in our brain. The processes of angiogenesis, the formation of new blood vessels in our brain, and neuroangiogenesis, the formation of new nerve cells in our brain, are both stimulated by exercise. This is thought to contribute to the prevention of cognitive decline as we age.

Exercise also decreases our risk of stroke and leads to an increase in the presence of BDNF, or brain-derived neurotrophic factor, which is often called fertiliser or Miracle-Gro for the brain. BDNF helps develop stronger connections between brain neurons and makes them more effective, leading to improved cognition and improved mood. Research suggests that the number-one way to increase BDNF in our brain is through physical activity.

When it comes to sleep, research shows that thirty minutes of exercise five times a week results in a 65% reduction in sleeplessness. Exercise is seen as the number-one nonpharmaceutical alternative to sleeping tablets when it comes to improving the quality of our sleep.

Harvard lecturer Tal Ben-Shahar describes not exercising as being like taking a depressant. We all know what an antidepressant is. In contrast, a depressant would be a tablet you take to cause you to become depressed! He says that if we don't exercise and physically move our body, we may as well be wilfully taking a depressant. One study showed that the positive effect on the moods of participants from exercising was equivalent to taking an antidepressant over a period of six months, and that the cohort of patients who used exercise as their intervention rather that an antidepressant had a 30% decrease in relapse rates over the period of the next two years.[7]

If we were to compare exercise to a medication, imagine a pharmaceutical company launching a new blockbuster treatment that could achieve a reduction in the occurrence of type 2 diabetes, coronary heart disease, stroke, high blood pressure, breast cancer, colon cancer, osteoporosis, and obesity and reduce the incidence of all causes of mortality. It would surely be a multibillion-euro global bestseller! Remarkably, this is exactly what exercise can do for us.

Another often overlooked benefit of exercise is its ability to reduce stress. Stress occurs when the demands placed on us exceed our resources to handle them. Essentially, there is an imbalance, something happens, and we feel we're not able to cope with it, whether it's work related, a difficult relationship, financial issues, or whatever the case may be. It's a reasonable question to ask how exercise could be of benefit in such scenarios.

Stressful events activate our fight-or-flight stress response. This is a protective mechanism that allowed our ancestors to immediately prepare to fight or flee from danger, usually an attack by a lion, tiger, or other predator. The automatic fight-or-flight response prepared our body to flee from danger or to fight danger. It is mediated in our body by the release of adrenaline and cortisol, which produces drastic changes in our physiology. Typically, we would then either fight or flee from our attacker, and in so doing we use up the adrenaline and cortisol, allowing our bodies to reset back to baseline.

In the modern age, thankfully, our lives are rarely in danger, yet the same fight-or-flight response is activated by today's low-grade stressors, such as finances, traffic, a busy work environment, technology issues, and so forth. As a result, adrenaline and cortisol are still being produced, but because we don't have to fight or flee, they aren't used up and so continue to circulate in our body. We call this chronic stress, and over the long term, these hormones produce damage that leads to various health problems and conditions.

Where exercise has been shown to be beneficial is that it allows us to use up these hormones and essentially sweat them out of our body. We call this completing the stress cycle. This is the mechanism by which exercise improves our ability to counteract stress and makes us more resilient. Of course, we have many different tools to cope with stress, including breath work, meditation, and cognitive behavioural therapy techniques. Exercise is a highly practical tool whereby we use our physical bodies to counteract stress.

Armed with this knowledge of the extensive benefits of moving our body on a regular basis, the next and most crucial step is to take committed, regular action. To assist with that, here are nine simple strategies to help you move your body more on a regular basis.

9 Tips to Get Moving

1. **Mindset Matters:** The hotel maid study, led by psychologist Ellen Langer, explored how mindset impacts health. Researchers told one group of hotel maids that their daily work, like vacuuming and scrubbing, met the U.S. Surgeon General's criteria for an active lifestyle. A control group received no such information. After four weeks, despite no change in actual behavior, the informed maids experienced significant improvements in weight, blood pressure, body fat, and BMI. This study highlighted the power of perception. Simply viewing their work as exercise led to real physiological benefits, showing that beliefs can directly influence wellbeing. This suggests a placebo effect or an expectation effect when it comes to our views around movement and exercise. Mindset, it seems, truly matters.

2. **Create Joyful Movement:** The more your movement is joyful and something that you really enjoy, the more likely you are to continue it. One of the two

easiest ways to make an activity more enjoyable is to exercise as part of a group. This not only creates accountability but also assists in building social connections and deepening relationships. Secondly, enjoyment increases when we exercise in natural surroundings, sometimes called blue-green exercise.

3. **The Seven-Minute Rule:** This is beneficial as a way to fool ourselves into exercising. At times we may feel we're not able to work up the energy to exercise, and with the seven-minute rule, we commit to exercising for just seven minutes. If, after the seven minutes have elapsed, we aren't enjoying ourselves, we simply stop. More often than not, however, what happens is that once we start, we feel like continuing. Once an object is in motion, it is more likely to stay in motion. The reason for this is that often it's the thought of the exercise rather than the exercise itself that is the deterrent, and we actually enjoy moving our bodies far more in the moment than we estimate in advance.

4. **NEAT Exercise:** This stands for non-exercise activity thermogenesis and is just the energy expended that isn't used for sleeping, eating, sports, or exercise. It is the energy we use going about our daily business, such as walking to work, doing the shopping, cleaning the house, and weeding the garden. Remember, all physical activity counts as exercise, and we don't actually have to be togged out in our exercise gear to

move our body. As already mentioned, modern life is hyperfocused on convenience, and so we have to find ways to reengineer movement back into our lives.

5. **Eliminate Perfection:** On many occasions we don't take up a new activity because we think we would look foolish or we would stand out and not be as adept at the activity as others. We wouldn't know what to do or where to start. It's important to remember that everyone started at the beginning and that the only difference between you and an expert is that they started before you.

6. **The Power Of 1% Gains:** We don't have to make massive changes in our lives to make a difference. Small changes that are sustainable are very beneficial and, in fact, are the only thing that really make a difference in the long run; that five-minute stretch in the morning, or a walk down the road for five minutes, then turning, and all of a sudden you have a ten-minute walk completed. Ultimately 1% gains, translates into huge improvements over time. When it comes to the benefits of movement, many of these accrue to us not necessarily based on our level of fitness but on the simple fact that we move our body.

7. **Be Firm But Compassionate:** Sometimes we berate ourselves about the gym session we missed or the run we didn't go for and end up giving out to ourselves for not being more disciplined. We think that being hard

on ourselves is a successful way to motivate ourselves, but in reality, it just makes us feel bad. This results in our exercise routine becoming just another stressor in our life, another thing to beat ourselves up about. It is helpful to reframe exercise as a gift we get to give ourselves rather than something we have to do. As a result, we interface with our exercise in a more compassionate way. This is not to say we constantly let ourselves off the hook for not exercising, so we need to find a balance between being compassionate and being firm.

8. **Exercise Early:** For those who are using exercise as a means to boost mood, it is more beneficial to exercise early in the morning. One study not only showed that college students showed a mood boost twenty minutes after exercise but also found that their moods were elevated two hours, four hours, eight hours, and even up to twelve hours later.[8] As a result, when we exercise in the evening, we may not experience the full benefits in terms of our mood.

9. **Measurement Creates Improvement:** One of the secrets of medicine is that measurement creates improvement. It has long been known that if you ask people to track an outcome, they are more likely to improve that outcome. For example, if you go to a dietician or nutritionist, the first thing you'll be asked to do is keep a food diary. It's similar when you visit your doctor if you are concerned about your blood pressure.

When we begin to track variables, we automatically receive a boost or improvement, whether that be in terms of foods consumed, steps taken, or blood pressure scores. Because of this phenomenon, it's a good idea to set a goal for your daily activity. Whether that be ten thousand steps or whatever is appropriate based on your current level of activity, the act of actively measuring a metric leads to improvements.

People often ask how much exercise they should try to fit into their weekly schedule. A commonsense approach is to get as much movement as you realistically can, knowing that more is better than some and some is better than none. Variety is also key, not only to prevent boredom but also to work on the various aspects of physical fitness; namely, cardiovascular, resistance, and flexibility.

Story: Sharpen Your Axe

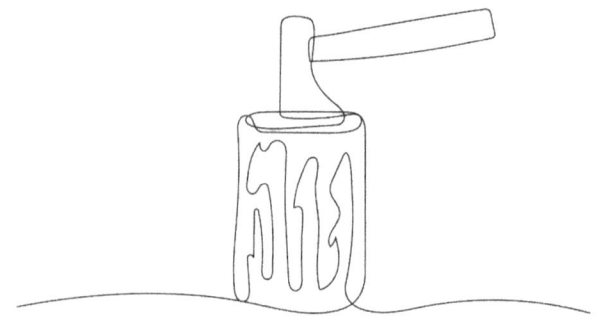

Once upon a time, there were two woodcutters, named Peter and Paul, who lived in the same town. Both were very competitive, and so they decided to hold a woodcutting competition: Whoever produced the most wood in one day would be the winner. Early that morning they both rose at dawn and started cutting away trees at the fastest possible speed.

Chop, chop, chop . . . The sound of axes hitting wood echoed throughout the forest, and both contestants matched their opponent stroke for stroke. This lasted for an hour, and all of a sudden Peter stopped. When Paul noticed there was no chopping, he thought Peter must be tired already, and so he continued to chop down his trees with double the motivation and at double the pace.

A quarter of an hour passed, and Paul heard his opponent chopping again. Once again after an hour, Peter stopped chopping. Feeling motivated and sensing victory close by, Paul continued on. Fifteen minutes later, Paul could hear the chopping sound again.

This went on the whole day. Every hour Peter would stop chopping the wood for fifteen minutes while Paul kept going persistently. Paul was totally confident that he would triumph. But to Paul's surprise, at the end of the day, Peter had actually chopped down more wood.

'I heard you stop working every hour for fifteen minutes!' Paul exclaimed. *'How could you possibly have cut more wood than me?'*

'*I was sharpening my axe,*' Peter replied.

In life, everybody, everywhere seems to be busy, running, racing, and chasing, caught up on the treadmill of life, dealing with the daily issues that arise. Most people are just too busy doing and don't spare the essential time required to rest, renew, and rejuvenate, to learn and grow; to '*sharpen the axe.*' To meet targets and deadlines, we work hard continuously. We feel exhausted and drained, and our effectiveness and productivity suffer. And it's simply not enough to take a break, relax, and rest. This isn't sharpening the axe; it's just putting the axe down. The blade will still be blunt. We need a balanced strategy to renew ourselves physically, mentally, emotionally, and spiritually. We need to be mindful of our diet, sleep, and exercise, to make meaningful connections with friends and family, to spend time in nature, to meditate.

CHAPTER 4

Discover and Apply Your Strengths

Tool: Strengths Awareness and Use
Pillar: Achievement

Nerves that fire together, wire together.
—Donald Hebb

Discovering Strengths to Boost Wellbeing

Next, we arrive at the A in the REVAMP model, which stands for Achievement. Identifying and applying our personal strengths significantly increases the likelihood of achieving our goals and serves as a powerful way to enhance wellbeing. When we actively use our strengths, we feel more engaged and connected to our lives because these strengths reflect our authentic selves.

To get the most out of this chapter, it is recommended to complete the free character strengths survey available at www.viacharacter.org. The survey is a quick process, taking just ten to fifteen minutes, and provides a ranked list of 24 character strengths that are universal to humanity. This survey has been taken by millions of individuals worldwide, and hundreds of research studies have shown the positive impact of applying our strengths in various areas of life.

The first step is to get to know what our strengths are, and the second is to consciously find ways to use these strengths in our daily lives. Strengths have applications across the entire spectrum of our lives, including our career, family, sports participation and coaching, education, goal setting, and recovery from illness.

So what are strengths, and why should we care? As human beings we tend to have a negativity bias, which is our tendency to notice the bad, the problems, the threats, the mistakes, and all the difficulties in our lives. We can describe our brains as being like Teflon for the good and Velcro for the bad when it comes to noticing our thoughts. Bad stuff is really attention grabbing for our brains, and negative thoughts are more likely to linger. We tend to dwell on and focus on the negative. Even though there's good stuff happening all around us every single minute of every single day, we don't tend to focus on it, and when we do, we discount it. This is true not only for the way we view the world but also for the way we view ourselves.

When I ask clients to tell me a little bit about their weaknesses, in general, I find they can describe what they're not good at in great detail. They then go on to tell me about all the things they wish they were better at, and how embarrassed they are about perceived weaknesses, and the consequences those weaknesses have had in their lives. When I then ask them to tell me a little about their strengths, I'm usually met with silence! It's as if they have never even considered strengths in themselves, as if they don't even fully understand the question. A Google Scholar search reinforces this bias, as we find lots of results, articles, and terminology to describe flaws, faults, and failings but far fewer describing our strengths and what we are good at. Lots of results for anxiety, less for joy. Lots for depression, less for happiness. This reveals a natural bias in humans to focus on weaknesses and flaws in ourselves, an extension of our negativity bias.

Two of the founding fathers of positive psychology, Martin Seligman and Chris Peterson, were really bothered by this imbalance. Martin Seligman, in his inauguration speech on becoming president of the American Psychological Association in 1998 described psychology as a half-baked cake.[9] He noted how psychology seemed to be obsessed with sickness, illness, and disorder, focusing almost exclusively on what goes wrong. Psychology deals with what's wrong, what's broken, what's diseased, and how we can fix it. He asked how we can show people how to boost their levels of wellbeing, how we can show them how to flourish or thrive in their lives, if we don't even have the words, language, or vocabulary to describe what that looks like? And so Chris Peterson and Martin Seligman set about correcting that imbalance.

The Diagnostic and Statistical Manual of Mental Disorders (DSM) serves as a universal reference for identifying and treating mental illnesses. It offers a standardised framework that enables doctors, whether in Ireland, Australia, or America, to effectively communicate about symptoms, diagnoses, and treatments.

Inspired to take an alternative approach, Martin Seligman and Chris Peterson created what they referred to as the Anti-DSM to provide a reference guide that celebrates strengths, wellbeing, and what is positive and strong in individuals, and thus helping to advance the understanding of human flourishing.

In 2004 they undertook a global study that reached every corner of the world, studying various cultures, nations, and societies. They examined literature, poetry, drama, media, politics, and sports and wrote a book called *Character Strengths and Virtues*, which describes twenty-four characteristics that are common to all of humanity. With the advent of the internet, this book morphed into the www.viacharacter.org website and online survey.

List of Twenty-Four Strengths

Appreciation of Beauty & Excellence	Gratitude	Kindness	Prudence
Bravery	Honesty	Leadership	Self-Regulation
Creativity	Hope	Love	Social Intelligence
Curiosity	Humility	Love of Learning	Spirituality
Fairness	Humour	Perseverance	Teamwork
Forgiveness	Judgement	Perspective	Zest

Unlocking the Power of Strengths for Wellbeing

The twenty-four strengths identified by Seligman and Peterson possess unique and deeply impactful characteristics. These strengths are universal, meaning they resonate across cultures and societies, uniting humanity through shared values. Importantly, they are also inherently rewarding to use. Engaging with our strengths feels fulfilling and uplifting, creating a sense of genuine enjoyment and purpose.

These strengths aren't just random abilities; they are qualities that positively contribute to humanity. For instance, while mastering table tennis is an admirable skill, it doesn't necessarily benefit humanity in the way that kindness, curiosity, or perseverance might! What makes these strengths even more remarkable is their ability to grow, and we can cultivate, nurture, and enhance them in ourselves over time.

At its core, a strength is a combination of something we excel at and truly enjoy doing. When we tap into our strengths:

- **We feel energised and excited:** Using our strengths naturally feels rewarding.
- **We experience increased engagement:** They help us feel deeply connected to what we are doing.
- **We feel authentically ourselves:** Our strengths reveal what is most true and admirable about us.

Ever heard of being 'in the zone?' That state of complete immersion where time seems to vanish and your focus sharpens? Using our character strengths is one of the best ways to access this state, often referred to as 'flow.' When we're in this state, life feels deeply meaningful, and our wellbeing soars.

Think of your character strengths as your personal superpowers. They align with your authentic self and enable you to contribute uniquely to the world. By using them, you shine, not just in your personal life but also in your interactions with others. And here's the best part. All strengths are buildable. Whether it's courage, creativity, or gratitude, you can actively work on enhancing them to elevate your life.

Start by identifying the strengths you use most often and notice how they light you up. Reflect on moments when you've felt completely yourself and at your best.

Those moments probably involved one or more of your core strengths.

Remember, strengths aren't just what you're good at; they are what make life meaningful and vibrant. By weaving them into your daily life, you create opportunities for growth, joy, and a deeper sense of wellbeing.

Strengths Focus

We all possess strengths but don't always focus on them. Our friends, family, and colleagues have strengths too, but we often fixate on faults or failings, in ourselves and others. However, if I ask you to think of someone such as a friend, family member, or colleague who is a real people's person, I'm sure you could readily do so. Perhaps they are a great communicator, loving to engage with friends, clients, or customers. If there's anyone likely to organise a social event or group weekend away, it's this person. Their natural inclination towards others represents the strength of social intelligence

Similarly, if you think about a colleague who is excellent at organising, setting up systems, and paying attention to detail, you'd likely have someone in mind. This person, who ensures all their t's are crossed and i's dotted, demonstrates the strength of appreciation of excellence. The same applies to traits like leadership, teamwork, creativity, perseverance, and more. Recognising and appreciating these strengths enables us to celebrate what makes people truly exceptional.

Our strengths are like the blueprints of how our brain operates at its absolute best. You've likely heard the saying, 'Nerves that fire together wire together.' This refers to the way our brain strengthens its pathways through repetition of thoughts or actions. Every time you think a certain thought or complete a specific action, a message travels through a neural pathway in your brain. The more you repeat it, the stronger and more defined that pathway becomes.

It's like skiing down a mountain after a fresh snowfall. The first ski run leaves tracks, but as you return and ski down the same path, the grooves in the snow deepen, smooth out, and make future runs faster and more automatic. The same principle applies to our strengths. Over time, we've formed robust neural pathways for our natural strengths, making them feel effortless and second nature. This ingrained efficiency is why using our strengths feels so satisfying and aligned with who we are.

Think of an experienced London cabbie who could drive from any point A to point B in London without the use of a map. On examination, their brains have denser fibres in the area responsible for spatial awareness. Or consider a concert pianist, who would have denser fibres in the area of their brain responsible for fine motor movement. This is referred to as neuroplasticity, wherein our brain changes and adapts to the demands placed on it. The same occurs with our strengths; our brains have adapted so that their use feel natural and effortless and simply flows out of us.

To illustrate this point, I'd like you to complete the following exercise.

Exercise

Place a pen in your dominant hand and write your first name and surname.
Then switch the pen to your nondominant hand, and once again write your first name and surname.
Notice how different it feels to write with each hand.

What people tend to notice from this exercise is that writing with their nondominant hand is effortful, feels unnatural and abnormal, and gives less-than-perfect results. In contrast, writing with one's dominant hand is effortless, natural, takes little thought, and yields perfect results. When you use your dominant hand, the process is completely automatic and ingrained. It simply flows out of you. You've repeated this same action countless times for years, decades even. As a result, you don't have to think about it. You could literally do it in your sleep, and you could certainly do it with your eyes closed.

That is really similar to how it feels when we're using our strengths. When we use our strengths, we often feel deeply engaged and in the zone, or what's often referred to as being 'in the flow.' This state of engagement not only makes us more productive but also enhances our sense of satisfaction in life. Simply put, focusing on our strengths allows us to achieve more with less effort, and in doing so, it boosts our wellbeing immeasurably.

One of the most exciting aspects of strengths is their potential for growth. The aren't fixed traits. Even if a particular strength doesn't come naturally to you, it's entirely possible to build and refine it using specific tools, practical techniques, and mindset adjustments. Imagine turning one of your weaknesses into a skill that energises and supports your goals.

See your strengths as multipliers for success. Not only do they help you achieve your goals with ease, but they also represent the best parts of you. It isn't just about achieving outcomes; it's about unlocking who you are at your core.

And here's the best part: using your strengths is inherently satisfying. It's energising. It feels right because it aligns with the essence of how you're naturally wired to thrive.

We can take social intelligence as an example. Those who score high on the strength of social intelligence love interacting and communicating with people. In a work scenario, they will thrive in an environment where they interact with others, maybe in a customer-facing role or as part of a team as opposed to being isolated and alone in an office at the back of a building. Similarly, someone who has a love of learning as their top strength will be stimulated and fulfilled by researching products, understanding the mechanics of a service or product, and understanding and getting into all the finer details and nitty-gritty. They may have no interest in interacting with others but prefer to have their head buried in research. We all have our own particular strengths, and the more we get to use them on a daily basis, the more energised and engaged in our lives we will be.

How do we go about incorporating strengths into our daily lives? The very first step is to find out what our strengths are. The next step is to find opportunities to use them. This creates a win-win situation, because as individuals, we benefit from applying the very best of us, but also at an organisational level, there are obvious benefits when everyone is using their strengths on a regular basis.

What is fascinating is that many people don't have any knowledge of what their strengths are. There are a couple of reasons for this. Firstly, as already mentioned, we have a negativity bias, which predisposes our brains to look for all our faults and failings rather than what's good, what's working, and what's strong about us. Secondly, we don't really have the language or vocabulary to describe what's great about us. Thirdly, there's also a cultural issue, in that it may be seen as being a bit arrogant to talk about our strengths. Finally, and perhaps most interestingly, is that we all suffer from a phenomenon called '*strengths blindness*,' where our strengths are so inherent to us, and are so much an expression of our true selves, that they just flow out of us and we don't even recognise them as being strengths.

For example, imagine your top strength is kindness and you're walking down the road with a friend when you see someone in difficulty and in need of assistance. Your natural inclination is to go and do whatever you can to help that person. Afterwards, your friend might comment on how kind and compassionate you were in that situation, but maybe you don't really see it like that, because for you it was the most normal and natural thing to do to help another human being in distress. That is the blindness we have, where something is so normal to us that we assume everyone sees and approaches things the way we would. This is not to suggest you are any better or worse than others, merely that you have a particular focus, a particular strength.

Signature Strengths

The VIA survey ranks twenty-four strengths that are universally present in humans. On completion of the survey, the first step is to look at your top five strengths. These are called your signature strengths. They are the very, very essence of who you are as a human being. They are central to you, but you may take them for granted. They feel so natural to you that they are energising, engaging, and exciting to use. If you get nothing else from this chapter, at the very least you now have a list of words that describe what is right about you. Research shows that if we are even aware of our strengths, and if we can name them from memory; we are more likely to experience high levels of wellbeing. If we get an opportunity to use our strengths on a daily basis, we are eighteen times more likely to experience high wellbeing.

When we know someone's top strengths, it gives us a window into their values, interests, and passions. I remember the first time I did the VIA strengths survey and I saw that appreciation of beauty and excellence was my top strength. I was somewhat disappointed! I didn't really see the value in appreciation of beauty and excellence when it came to my future career. I imagined a future employer asking me in an interview about my top strengths and replying that I was really good at appreciating beauty! However, when I became more familiar with the language, terminology, and vocabulary of strengths, it became clearer to me how this strength showed up in my life.

For many years I have really loved running. It's just my thing; it energises me and elevates my mood. However, I refuse to run on the road and love nothing more than to run in a forest, a field, by the sea, by a lake, or up the mountains. Give me a day off and that's where I'm going, no question. I can't fully explain it, I don't know what happens to me, but I just get completely absorbed by running in nature. I feel inspired, elevated, and energetic, so much so that I often feel like I could just go on forever. That's an expression of an appreciation of beauty and how it shows up in my life. The appreciation of excellence element is also obvious in my work as a pharmacist. I love order, systems, checkboxes, and procedures. I love to have an efficient system where everyone knows what to do to ensure we perform at a high standard. I get stressed when there is disorder, chaos, and untidiness. It is important to me that we provide a consistent level of excellent customer service.

I also really admire and am fascinated by people who are at the top of their game in sports, business, and life. All of the above are examples of how an appreciation for beauty and excellence show up in my life. When we know someone's strengths, it gives us insight into how they view the world, their values, their passions, and their interests. This enables us to get to know someone through the lens of what's right about them rather than focusing on their faults and failings. Spotting strengths in others can completely change relationships. All it takes is a level of awareness and some practice. A good place to start is to think of prominent figures in society and identify their strengths, what makes them exceptional.

When we think of Albert Einstein, we think of curiosity, love of learning, humour. Mother Teresa brings to mind kindness and compassion. The Dalai Lama has the obvious strengths of humility, perseverance, serenity, and compassion.

With practice, strengths can become a beautiful lens through which we view others. This is the real power of a strengths focus; it changes how we look at others so that rather than being suspicious, cynical, or wary of people, we purposefully look for their strengths in our interactions with them. Imagine the difference this could make to your relationships with your partner, your children, your friends, and your work colleagues.

Do you think it would be useful to know the strengths of your partner? Imagine knowing exactly how they view the world, their perspective, their outlook, and how their brain is wired to perform at its very best. How might it positively influence your relationship if you knew what their strengths were and every time you spotted them being used, you let them know? Getting into the habit of validating someone, recognising the very best parts of them and letting them know every time you see them using one of their strengths, can be truly transformational for a relationship. Sometimes our default can be to do the exact opposite, to point out their every fault and failing and let them know all the things they should improve about themselves. For example, if your partner's top strength is bravery, imagine how wonderful it would feel for them if you acknowledged every time you saw them using it: *'I know it was really hard for you to speak up in that situation, but I really admire your bravery in doing so.'* Or if their top strength is perseverance: *'I know you're going through a really tough time at the moment, and every day I see how you persevere. I really admire that about you.'*

The same is true when it comes to the strengths of our children. Oftentimes, the difficult teenage years can be full of conflict, misunderstanding, and poor communication. Viewing your teen through the lens of strengths can also be transformational, as it gives you as a parent many opportunities to spot your teen doing something right rather than having all your conversations be negative and critical of them.

Using Strengths for Better Communication

Knowing the strengths of someone you have challenges with can also lead to improvements in communication and understanding. Many times when we have challenges with people, it's just because we have a vastly different picture of the world and view things completely differently. Essentially, our differences can stem from a collision of our strengths. If we have insight into the lens through which they view the world by being aware of their strengths, it can help us to reframe our relationship.

A good example of this would be two work colleagues on the same team, one with the strength of creativity and the other with the strength of prudence. The creative person's focus is on considering new and innovative concepts in relation to a product or service. They may no sooner have come up with a novel approach than they immediately move on to another idea. You can imagine how this approach would clash with that of someone whose top strength is prudence.

Awareness and consistent use of your strengths have a profound impact on your wellbeing. They help you feel energised, engaged, and more productive in your daily life. When we have the opportunity to use our strengths regularly, it enhances not only our performance but also our sense of fulfilment. For example, if your top strength is social connection, could you reshape your role to include more interpersonal interactions? This might involve participating in customer service initiatives, helping with onboarding new recruits, or fostering teamwork and collaboration within your team. Similarly, if leadership is one of your key strengths, you might consider engaging in leadership development programmes, becoming a mentor for junior colleagues, or finding ways to inspire and positively influence others. It's also important to recognise that our strengths are not confined to specific contexts or domains. For instance, you may notice you consistently apply one of your signature strengths in one area of your life, such as work, but not in another, like at home or in your community. Reflecting on and intentionally applying your strengths across different facets of your life can create a more balanced and thriving existence.

A personal example of this for me is humour, which is one of my top five strengths. When I took the time to reflect on how humour showed up in my life, I realised that while I often used it in my personal life with friends and family, I avoided it entirely at work. Being the boss, I felt that using humour with my team might undermine my authority or lead them to take me less seriously. However, after some thought, I recognised that by suppressing this aspect of my personality at work, I wasn't being authentic, and consequently, I didn't feel as relaxed around my colleagues. This prompted me to make a change. I decided to bring humour into my professional interactions in a thoughtful and appropriate way. Since making this shift, my team has gained a deeper understanding of who I am, and I feel more genuine and at ease in the workplace. It's been a positive change for everyone involved, fostering a more open and engaging work environment.

It is a great idea to ask yourself *Where in my life am I not using my strengths on a regular basis?* For example, if my top strength is leadership and I use that frequently at work, could I also use it in my local youth sports club or in a community initiative? This would benefit not only my community but also me, because when I use my strengths, I feel engaged, energised, and fulfilled.

Another important consideration when it comes to strengths is the balance in how we express them. Strengths are most effective when they are displayed in what we might call the Goldilocks sweet spot. Not too much, not too little, but just right. Take honesty, for example. It's a wonderful strength to possess, but if overused, it can come across as bluntness or even insensitivity. Similarly, humour can bring joy and connection, yet if used inappropriately or at the wrong time, it might come off as buffoonery. Excess bravery, while admirable, could lead to reckless risk-taking and appear foolhardy. To make the most of our strengths, it's essential to strike the right balance to harness their full potential without causing unintended consequences.

One simple idea for incorporating strengths into our daily life includes picking one task on our to-do list and asking ourselves *How can I use a strength to complete this task?* Then we simply pick the most appropriate of our strengths and write it down beside the task. For example, we might decide;

- *In this afternoons meeting, I will use my strength of fairness to ensure my feelings don't bias my decisions,*
- *or I will use my strength of curiosity to solve the challenge my team is facing,*
- *or I will call on my strength of perseverance to ensure I complete my training program for the upcoming marathon.*

One powerful mindset to adopt is putting on your 'strengths goggles.' Imagine viewing everyone you meet through a lens that highlights their strengths; their unique qualities that are good, right, and admirable. This perspective shift can transform relationships, fostering deeper understanding and appreciation. It challenges us to consciously seek out and focus on the best in others, creating connections rooted in positivity and respect.

To begin, start by identifying your own top five signature strengths. Write them down, take time to explore them, and bring them to the forefront of your awareness. By recognising and appreciating these strengths in yourself, you'll be better equipped to spot and nurture them in others, ultimately inspiring a more meaningful connection with those around you.

Story: The Teacher's Mistake

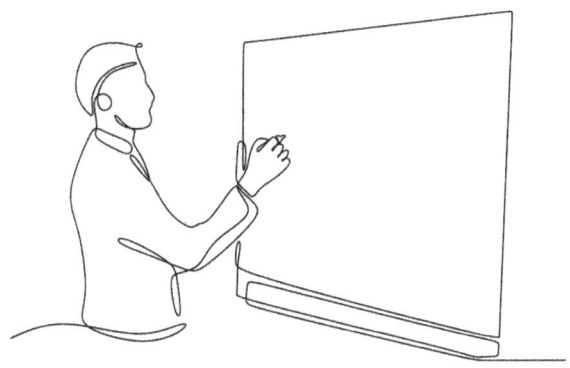

One morning in a busy classroom, the teacher wrote a sequence of maths equations on the board:
As soon as he was finished and stepped aside, the room filled with giggles and whispers. Finally, one student raised their hand and said, '*Sir, you made a mistake. The last equation is wrong. Five times five is twenty-five, not twenty-six.*'

The teacher nodded and smiled as he looked around the classroom, his eyes scanning the students. '*You're absolutely right. I did make a mistake. But here is a question for all of you. Did anyone notice that I got the first four equations right?*' The class fell silent, the giggles and laughter fading into thought.

The teacher continued. '*This is a lesson for life. Too often we focus on mistakes and weakness, overlooking strengths and success. The world will often highlight what you do wrong, but it's your job to focus on what you've done right.*'

He walked around the room, letting the lesson sink in. *'If you focus only on your weakness, you'll feel deflated. But when you recognise your strengths, you'll build confidence in your abilities. The same applies to how you see others, and acknowledging their successes instead of just pointing out their flaws.'* Let this be a reminder your strengths deserve more attention than your flaws. When you focus on yourself and what you do well you see yourself differently.

CHAPTER 5

The Search for Meaning

Tool: Clarifying Values
Pillar: Meaning

Values are like fingerprints. Nobody's are the same, but you leave them all over everything you do.

—Elvis Presley

Next we move on to the M in the REVAMP model, representing Meaning. What is meaning, and why does it matter? In modern life where distractions are everywhere and expectations are high, the search for meaning is more relevant than ever. Whereas our happiness tends to come and go throughout life, meaning is stable and is what anchors us. It gives us a sense of purpose that persists even in life's most difficult moments.

Most of us will have asked ourselves at some point throughout life Why am I doing this? What is it all about? These questions often arise in times of difficulty, stress, or struggle. Maybe it's a job that no longer excites us, a relationship that has lost its sparkle, or a routine that has become boring. When we lack a strong sense of meaning, everything can begin to feel like a series of disconnected tasks, things we '*have to*' do rather than things we '*get to*' do.

Meaning isn't a luxury reserved for philosophers and poets but is a basic human need leading to higher life satisfaction, improved wellbeing, and even longer lifespans. In fact, research shows that having a sense of meaning and purpose reduces the risk of depression, lowers stress and anxiety, and improves overall resilience. Those who feel their lives have meaning are also more engaged in their work and relationships, and they are more motivated in their daily tasks.

It isn't something we just stumble on but is something we cultivate and grow through the stories we tell ourselves, the values we hold, and the contributions we make to others.

Cultivating a greater sense of meaning in our lives has three key elements: coherence, purpose, and significance.

Coherence

Coherence is how we make sense of the story of our life and begins with understanding our own story. Life is full of ups and downs, unexpected twists, and difficult challenges. It's in how we interpret these experiences that meaning is created. Writer Isabel Allende once said, *'You are the storyteller of your own life, and you can create your own legend or not.'* If we see our struggles as meaningless obstacles, they can feel overwhelming. However, if we frame them as necessary steps in our journey, they become part of a larger, purposeful story. Think of a time when you faced a challenge. When you reflect on it, ask yourself whether it led to personal growth, a new opportunity, or deepening of a relationship. When we find patterns and lessons in our experiences, we create coherence. The sense that our lives make sense, even when they don't go as planned.

> ### *Exercise*
>
> Think of a significant challenge you have overcome. How did it shape the person you have become? How did you grow and develop as a result? How does this challenge fit into the bigger story of your life?

Purpose

Purpose is the driving force that moves us forward. It is about aligning our actions with our personal values, ensuring we invest our time and energy into what really matters. It's what motivates us to out of bed in the morning. Contrary to what we are often led to believe, finding purpose is not about discovering some grand, life-changing mission. It's about engaging in activities that resonate with who we actually are. Purpose evolves with us and is dynamic, not static. For some, it may be found in their work, while for others it may be found in parenting, volunteering, or engaging in creative pursuits. The key is to regularly ask ourselves whether we're spending our time on what truly matters to us.

Exercise

What activities energise and inspire you?
When do you feel most engaged and alive?
How can you bring your values more into your daily life?

Significance

Significance is the sense that we are contributing to something bigger than ourselves, and making a difference in the world, creating a ripple effect that extends beyond us. There is a lovely saying: *What we do for ourselves dies with us. What we do for others and the world remains and is immortal.* Whether it's helping a friend, mentoring a colleague, or doing work that benefits our community, our actions ripple outward in ways we may never fully see or appreciate.

> *Exercise*
>
> Think of a time you made a positive impact on someone's life.
> How did it make you feel?
> How can you incorporate more acts of contribution into your life on a daily basis?

Often we mistakenly believe that meaning is found in extraordinary achievements, but in reality it's the small, everyday moments that bring the deepest sense of fulfilment. One study asked participants to photograph what they found meaningful in their lives. The results clearly showed that meaning was most often found in relationships, small joys, and acts of kindness and compassion. Some people submitted images of family gatherings, handwritten letters from friends, or even a quiet walk in nature. Others found meaning in their work, a simple cup of tea shared with a friend, or the act of helping a stranger.

If you were to bring to mind the most meaningful moments of your life, what would you include? Who are the people, places, and experiences that give your life a sense of meaning and purpose?

In the modern world it is not uncommon for us to spend our days rushing from task to task, crossing items off our never-ending to-do lists yet still feeling empty at the end of the day. Busyness does not equal fulfilment. If our daily actions don't align with our values, we risk suffering from burnout, disengagement, and dissatisfaction.

The Role of Values

The connection between values and meaning is powerful. When we align our actions with what matters most to us, our lives feel richer, more purposeful, and more rewarding. By getting clear on our values, then living our lives in accordance with them, we strengthen our sense of authenticity and create a sense of coherence in our life's story.

Values are more than abstract ideas; they are the foundation of a meaningful life. Each day, every decision gives us an opportunity to reinforce our values and leave an imprint that is true to who we are. Values become a compass that guides our decisions, clarifies our priorities, and connects us with our sense of meaning. When we align our actions with our personal values, we connect to a sense of meaning and fulfilment that boosts our wellbeing. On the other hand, when we ignore our values, life can seem disconnected and shallow.

This connection between values and meaning allows us to make conscious choices that enhance our sense of purpose, improve relationships, and bring greater clarity to the life we are trying to build.

So what exactly are values? Values are our deep beliefs that influence how we see the world and what we view as important. They are the standards that guide how we act and behave, shape our decisions, and help us determine what is worthwhile. They are often shaped by our upbringing, culture, and personal experience. As we grow and evolve, so too do our values shift and change.

Common examples of values include:

- Integrity: Acting honestly and consistently with your beliefs.
- Compassion: Caring for others and showing empathy.

- Adventure: Seeking excitement, growth, and new experiences.
- Connection: Prioritising meaningful relationships with others.
- Creativity: Expressing originality and innovative thinking.

The key is to recognise which values matter most to us. By identifying these, we can create a road map for a more meaningful life. Values act as guiding principles that influence our goals, habits, and priorities. Without them we may drift aimlessly or pursue goals and objectives that fail to fulfil us. By understanding what we value most, we can make choices that align with those priorities, leading to a stronger sense of purpose.

For example, we may value connection and relationships but spend most of our time working overtime and neglecting our family and friends. Despite achieving success in our career, we may still feel unfulfilled. By realigning our lifestyle to prioritise relationships, we can rediscover a deeper sense of meaning.

The benefits of becoming familiar with our values include:

1. They create the sense that our life experiences form a consistent narrative that is essential to meaning. When our values guide our actions, we can connect past struggles, current efforts, and future goals into a coherent story.

2. Values inspire purpose, the feeling that what we do matters. When we act in alignment with our values, our daily routines take on new significance. Even mundane tasks can become purposeful when they connect to something greater.
3. They strengthen resilience. When we experience challenges, hardships, or uncertainty, values act as an anchor that grounds us. Research shows that individuals who can connect their difficulties to their values are better able to cope with adversity and maintain a sense of meaning.
4. Shared values play a crucial role in strengthening relationships. When people connect with others who prioritise similar principles, it fosters trust and enhances communication, creating a stronger bond.

Living in accordance with our values isn't always automatic but requires intention and practice. Here are some steps to ensure our actions reflect what matters most:

Exercise

1. Identify Your Values

Choose your five core values from the list of common personal values below.

Achievement	Gratitude	Nature	Simplicity
Balance	Health	Open-mindedness	Spirituality
Community	Honesty	Optimism	Success
Compassion	Humility	Patience	Sustainability
Courage	Independence	Peace	Teamwork
Dignity	Innovation	Perseverance	Tolerance
Empathy	Integrity	Quality	Tradition
Equality	Joy	Reliability	Transparency
Fairness	Kindness	Resilience	Trust
Family	Learning	Respect	Understanding
Freedom	Love	Responsibility	Wealth
Friendship	Loyalty	Security	Wisdom
Generosity	Mindfulness	Self-discipline	Work Ethic

It may be helpful to ask yourself:
What qualities do I admire most in others?
When have I felt most fulfilled and proud?
What principles am I not willing to compromise on?
Once you've identified your top five values, write them down and keep them visible so that you regularly bring them to mind.

2. Align Your Habits with Your Values
Once you know your values, assess your current routines. Do your daily actions reinforce them? For example, if you value connection, consider scheduling regular catch-ups with friends or dedicating more quality time to family. If you value learning, commit to reading one new book per month or listening to educational podcasts.

3. Set Value-Based Goals
Instead of setting goals based only on achievement, create goals that reflect your values. Value-driven goals provide deeper motivation and help ensure that success feels meaningful rather than empty. For example, if you value creativity, setting a goal to write a weekly blog or attend a painting class may feel far more fulfilling than setting an unrelated professional target.

4. Navigate Challenges with Values
When we're faced with difficult decisions, values offer us a clear guide for action. By aligning our responses with our top values, we are more likely to make choices that align with our identity and long-term fulfilment.

Finding Meaning in Work

For many of us, work takes up a significant portion of our lives. Studies show that people who find meaning in their work report greater job satisfaction, lower stress levels, and higher engagement. However, meaningful work doesn't just happen; we have to shape it.

The process of job crafting offers a very useful approach. It involves modifying our tasks, relationships, and mindset to align our work with our values and strengths, thus injecting it with more meaning. Small shifts, such as focusing on parts of our work that we enjoy, fostering deeper connections with colleagues, or finding purpose in how our work impacts others, can significantly enhance our sense of fulfilment.

Ask yourself the following questions:
- *What tasks in your work energise you, and which ones drain you?*

- *Are there small ways to shift your work to focus more on what excites you?*
- *How can you bring more of your true self, your values, interests, and strengths, to your role?*

Sometimes meaning isn't in the work itself but in how we approach it. A janitor at a hospital may see their job as simply cleaning floors, or they may see it as contributing to the healing environment for patients. Our perspective really matters.

Story: The Three Stonecutters

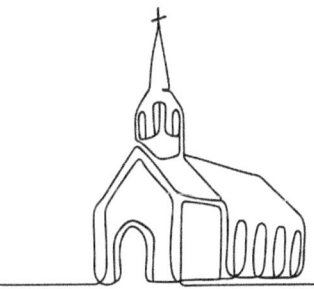

One day a traveller was passing through a small but busy town when he came upon a construction site. The place was filled with dust and noise, and the sharp sound of chisels striking stone echoed through the streets. Curious, the traveller approached the first worker he saw, a man hunched over a large slab of rock.

'*What are you doing?*' the traveller asked.

The man barely looked up, his face tired and sweat dripping from his forehead. '*I'm cutting stones,*' he muttered. '*It's backbreaking work, but I need the money. I do what I must to get by.*'

The traveller nodded and moved on, stopping at another stonecutter a few metres away. This worker had better posture and seemed more focused on his task. '*What about you?*' the traveller asked.

The man paused and put down his chisel. As he looked up, he said, '*I'm shaping these stones so they can fit together properly. We're building a wall,*' he explained. '*It's decent work, and I take pride in doing it well.*'

The traveller continued walking until he reached a third worker farther down the site. This man stood tall, working with energy and precision. There was something different about him, a sense of purpose in his movements. Intrigued, the traveller asked, '*And what about you? What are you doing?*'

The man looked up, his eyes full of enthusiasm. '*Ah,*' he said with a smile, '*I'm building a cathedral. One day, people will gather here to celebrate their lives' great moments. They will come to find peace, to reflect, to celebrate, and to connect with something bigger than themselves. Long after I'm gone, this place will stand as a symbol of hope and faith. My hands are shaping something that will matter for generations.*'

The traveller stood still for a moment, letting the words sink in. Three men, doing the same work, saw it in entirely different ways. One saw work, one saw a craft, and one saw a purpose.

Meaning isn't about what we do; it's about how we view it. Two people can perform the same task, but the one who connects it to something greater will always find deeper fulfilment. So ask yourself: In your work, in your life, are you just cutting stones? Or are you building something meaningful?

CHAPTER 6

The Power of Breath

Tool: Breath
Pillar: Positive Emotions

In a world of doing, doing, doing, it is important to breathe and just be.

—Stephanie Weber

The final pillar in the REVAMP model is P, which stands for Positive Emotions. Within the wellbeing community, there has been a growing emphasis on the power of the breath as a versatile and effective tool for enhancing overall wellbeing. Here, I would like to introduce you to a few safe, straightforward, and accessible techniques that are easy to implement. These methods avoid unnecessary complexity, steer clear of unrealistic medical claims, and do not promise mystical or supernatural outcomes. The breath is particularly fascinating in the context of the REVAMP model because it has the potential to support multiple pillars. By using the breath intentionally, we can influence our emotional state, deepen our sense of engagement, and boost our vitality, making it a truly powerful resource for enhancing positive emotions and overall resilience.

The Mechanics Of Breathing

At its most basic, breathing is about the exchange of gases. We inhale air, from which we extract oxygen, while excreting carbon dioxide when we exhale. This process takes place in our lungs. Our lungs are organs, not muscles. We have two lungs in our abdominal cavity, with our left lung being smaller than our right to accommodate our heart. The capacity of a man's lung is approximately 6 litres and that of a woman approximately 4.2 litres. The surface area of the interior of our lungs is often quoted as being similar to that of a tennis court, and this is important for facilitating extensive gaseous exchange as we breathe. It is said that when we consider all the tubes, tubules, airways, and branches of our lungs, if we place them end to end, they would extend to a distance of approximately two thousand kilometres!

The act of breathing is facilitated by a number of key muscles. Our diaphragm is an umbrella-shaped muscle that lies at the bottom of our rib cage beneath our lungs. When it contracts, it flattens, which has the effect of expanding our rib cage, creating a vacuum. This in turn has the effect of drawing air into the lungs to fill the vacuum. Importantly, the diaphragm consists of skeletal muscle, which is the same type of muscle found in our legs and arms, and means that the diaphragm can be toned, trained, and conditioned. Secondly, our intercostal muscles, which are located between our ribs, expand and lift our rib cage with each breath, and finally, the muscles of our neck, chest, shoulders, and back also facilitate the process of breathing.

At school we are usually taught that in breathing, oxygen is the good guy and carbon dioxide is the bad guy. However, both molecules have important roles to play in our body. Oxygen is required for energy production and is the spark that converts our food to energy. Oxygen is needed by every cell in our body. When we breathe in, the inhaled air contains approximately 21% oxygen, and when we exhale, the air contains approximately 14% oxygen. This shows us that it isn't a case of our bodies trying to hold on to every molecule of oxygen we can get, more a situation of an appropriate balance. Carbon dioxide, rather than just being a waste product, actually plays an important role in vasodilation, opening our breathing passageways and increasing oxygen absorption by our cells. It also performs a vital signalling function. The goal of breathing is to appropriately balance these two critical molecules in our body.

The Benefits Of Nasal Breathing

When we breathe, it is preferable to do so through our nose rather than our mouth, unless doing so is severely restricted by sinus, allergy, or nasal passage issues. Mouth breathing is associated with increased blood pressure, a faster pulse, sleep apnoea, and decreases in mental clarity. The nose has an important function in cleaning, heating, and moistening the air we take into our body. Native Americans compare breathing through the nose to drinking distilled water and breathing through the mouth to drinking poor-quality, contaminated water. In addition, when we breathe through our nose, we stimulate neuroreceptors at the top of our nostrils that send a signal to our brain that we are now safe and secure and that it's now appropriate for our body and mind to relax.

Nasal breathing also stimulates our sinuses to release nitric oxide, which acts as a vasodilator, expanding and relaxing the blood vessels and thus leading to improvements in circulation, increased uptake of oxygen by the cells, and improved immune function and mood. In fact, nitric oxide release increases sixfold, resulting in an 18% increase in oxygen absorption by simply breathing through our nose.

The mechanics of breathing are undoubtedly very interesting, but when we look at the breath on another level, a whole new world opens up to us. When we inhale air from our surroundings, we are, in fact, inhaling the very universe. More than just getting air into our body, breathing is the most intimate connection we can have with our surroundings. Every inhalation contains hand-me-down space dust that has been in existence for the last fourteen billion years, and so where our body begins and the universe ends becomes a blurred line. Again, at its most basic, breathing is about exchanging gases, but the breath plays a more subtle but equally powerful role.

Autonomic Nervous System

Our breath influences nearly every single internal organ and system, signalling it to either turn on or turn off, thus playing a role in our heart rate, digestion, and mood. All these effects are mediated by part of our nervous system called our autonomic nervous system, and this is where the breath becomes really interesting.

As detailed previously in the section about meditation, our autonomic nervous system is that part of our nervous system responsible for processes in our body that happen automatically and are not under our conscious control, such as our heart rate and digestion. Our autonomic system is divided into the sympathetic nervous system and the parasympathetic nervous system. The sympathetic nervous system is responsible for our stress response, also known as our fight-or-flight response, and the parasympathetic nervous system has an opposing effect and is all about rest, repair, and rejuvenation; calm, peace, and ease. Modern life throws these systems out of balance and reduces our ability to effectively transition between both necessary states. Typically, we get stuck in stress, worry, anxiety, and fear. The breath is the only connection between our conscious mind and our autonomic nervous system, and we can use the breath to quickly and effectively manipulate our emotional state.

Effectively influencing our emotional state is an integral part of daily life, whether we realise it or not. The concept of regulating our nervous system isn't new. It's something we naturally do every day. For instance, we often reach for caffeine or sugary treats to energise ourselves or elevate our mood temporarily. Similarly, we turn to Netflix marathons or a tub of Ben & Jerry's ice cream to relax and find a sense of calm. But what if there was a healthier and more sustainable way to achieve the same outcomes? By focusing on something as simple and accessible as our breath, we can regulate our emotional state in a balanced and intentional manner, avoiding the potential downsides of over-relying on these common coping mechanisms.

When it comes to using our breath consciously to alter our emotional state, there are a number of factors that we can use, namely, the depth, rate, and ratio of our breathing.

Long, slow, deep breaths through our nose are associated with calm, peace, and ease. The lower lobes of our lungs are adjacent to many parasympathetic nerve endings. Deep breaths stimulate these nerve endings and as a result send a signal to our body that we are safe and secure and that it is appropriate to turn on our rest-and-digest response.

On the other hand, there are lots of nerve endings associated with our sympathetic nervous system at the tops of our lungs, and consequently, short, sharp breaths stimulate these and act like an emergency call to our body's alert system.

The vagus nerve passes through the opening of the diaphragm and is the largest nerve in our parasympathetic nervous system. High vagal tone leads to improvements in many health outcomes, and low vagal tone is associated with poor cardiovascular health and an increased risk of stroke. The vagus nerve is stimulated by deep breathing, humming, singing, or chanting.

In general, breathing practices can be divided into three classes: stimulating, balancing, and relaxing. I refer to these classes as Sunrise, Balancing, and Sunset breaths.

Sunrise Breaths

Sunrise breaths are stimulating and energising. They help to activate us and are useful when it comes to achieving goals, preparing us for exercise, or invigorating us in the mornings. In modern-day life, except for these specific uses, we generally don't need too much help stimulating our sympathetic nervous system. As a result, these exercises are used moderately and are never pushed, as they can cause us to experience dizziness or overwhelm. An example of this class of exercise is Breath of Fire. In this breath practice we speed up breathing to approximately 30 breaths per minute.

Exercise – Breath of Fire

Begin in a seated position with eyes open or closed. Exhale fully through the nose by engaging the muscles of the abdomen, as if you were trying to touch your spine with your belly button.

This has the effect of creating a forceful exhalation, as if you were struck in the stomach by a football. After this sharp exhale, relax the abdomen and for the inhale simply allow the breath to enter through the nose.

The mouth remains closed throughout.

Continue at a quick pace of approximately 30 breaths per minute for a total of 20 breaths.

Then relax the breathing for 3-5 breaths and complete another two rounds of 20 breaths.

After completing the sequence, tune in to your body and notice an increase in your energy as you feel more alive, awake, and energised.

Balance Breaths

Balance breaths do exactly what they say on the tin! They are adaptogenic, meaning if we are stimulated, they can help to calm and soothe us, whereas if we are lethargic, they can energise us. An example of this class of exercise is the equal ratio breath. This exercise involves a slow five second inhale and a five second exhale. That pace gives us 6 breaths per minute. Inhale and exhale are the same length, in and out through the nose. There is just a moment of transition between inhale and exhale and exhale and inhale.

Exercise – Equal Ratio Breath

To start, take a deep clearing breath in and out through your mouth.
With your mouth closed, begin to slowly breathe in and out through the nose.
Each inhale should be close to 5 seconds long, with each exhale being of the same length.
Slowly, in 2, 3, 4, 5 followed by out 2, 3, 4, 5
Repeat this pattern for 3-5 minutes.
After completing the practice, tune in and note how you are feeling.

Sunset Breaths

Sunset breaths calm, soothe, and down-regulate us. Typically, we would perform these in the evening, in a lying-down position.

Exercise – Relaxing Breath

In a seated position, with eyes closed, bring your attention to your breath.
Place both hands on your stomach and feel it rising as you breathe in, and flatten as you breathe out.
Breathe in through your nose, breathe out through your nose.
Feel your stomach rising, stomach falling.
As you continue to breathe, notice your inhale.
Notice how long it is, and just to yourself slowly count out your inhalation..
So you might notice that it is the length of '1..2.. 3..4'
On your next breath double your exhale.
So if your inhale was to the count of 4 then now make your exhale to the count of 8.
It only has to be close - it doesn't have to be exact.

Continue breathing with your exhale doubled.
Notice how you feel, allowing your shoulders to drop on the out breath and feel your whole body relax.
Continue for 10 breaths and when you are ready open your eyes, tuning in to the sensation of relaxation and calm in your body and mind.

Some experts talk of the *'perfect breath'* as having an efficient rhythm with a 5.5-second inhale followed by a 5.5-second exhale, resulting in 5.5 breaths per minute. This breathing rate is thought to synchronise to many body rhythms. It has been observed that this pattern mimics the breathing pattern seen in the call and response of the rosary, and also resembles the breathing pattern produced by the *om* sound, which promotes a six-second *om*, followed by a six-second inhale.

Tongue in cheek, it has been said that *'prayer heals, especially at 5.5 breaths per minute.'* Breathwork has been described as *'meditation for those who don't want to meditate, yoga for those who don't want to get off the couch, and healing prayer for the nonreligious.'*

Story: The Calm Archer

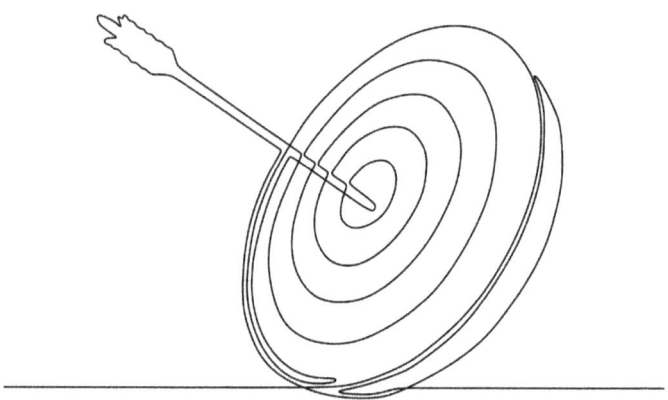

In a quiet village, a young boy watched the village archer with awe. The archer could hit any target, no matter how small or far away. One day the boy asked him, *'How do you stay so steady when you are in a competition and all eyes are focused on you?'*

The archer smiled and handed the boy his bow. *'Pull the string,'* he said, but as the boy pulled, his hand shook and the arrow missed the target. *'You see,'* the archer said, *'the bow cannot steady itself. It needs the archer to be calm. When you feel stress, fear, or anxiety, your breath is the first thing to change. But your breath is also the key to bringing your body back to stillness.'*

The archer took a long, slow, deep breath, and the boy watched as his body sank into stillness. *'Feel the rhythm of your breathing, and your body will soon follow. When your body is steady, your mind and emotions become clear, like a still pond reflecting the sky.'*

The boy practiced every day, learning to breathe deeply and anchor his body before releasing an arrow. Over time, he noticed that not only did his aim improve, but he also felt calmer, even when he was competing against others.

Years later, the young boy became the village's greatest archer, known for his skill with the bow, but more so for his unshakable calm. When asked for his secret, he would smile and say, *'The breath leads, the body follows, and the heart finds its way.'*

CHAPTER 7

Understanding Our Thoughts

Tool: Avoid Thinking Traps
Pillar: Positive Emotions

> *There are two ways to live your life. One is as though nothing is a miracle. The other is as though everything is a miracle.*
>
> —Albert Einstein

There are various tools and techniques available to us to boost all wellbeing pillars in the REVAMP model. Avoiding thinking traps is another useful intervention we can make to boost positive emotions. A key skill when it comes to improving wellbeing is the ability to recognise, experience, and, if necessary, alter our emotions. Emotions can be altered by focusing on and manipulating the way they are expressed in our brain, breath, and body, also known as the emotional triad.

The brain element of this triad refers to our thoughts. In this area we examine the nature of our self-talk; how we address ourselves and the tone, words, and focus we use. Here we look at, firstly, cultivating self-awareness, having the ability to hit the pause button and ask what thoughts we are having and whether they are helpful or harmful. This is important because our thoughts lead to our actions, which determine our results. Secondly, we look at self-regulation, having the ability to not just notice our thoughts but also to change them. This is called mental agility.

Thinking Traps

When we experience stress, anxiety, or worry, we often make errors in our logic and reasoning called cognitive distortions, also known as thinking traps. These are thought patterns that are inaccurate and unhelpful and make it hard to see a situation clearly. Thinking traps have some common triggers.

1. *Ambiguity.* This refers to when something is unclear or there is a degree of uncertainty. In these situations, our brain often fills in the gaps and more often than not defaults to a catastrophic, mostly negative interpretation. Examples of this would be when the boss comes into your office and says, '*We need to talk*,' or the doctor leaves a voice message saying, '*Call me;*

your results are back.' Both situations are ambiguous and so can trigger us to fall into a thinking trap.

2. *Higher value.* This refers to when something we perceive to be precious is at risk. For example, maybe your teenager was to be home by six p.m., and it's now nine p.m. and you have neither heard nor can get in contact with them. This may trigger worst case scenario thinking as we begin to spiral into worry.

3. *Fear.* The experience of fear or anxiety is likely to lead us to fall into a thinking trap. For example, if we have a fear of flying and we're about to get on board a plane, we are likely to catastrophise and have incessant illogical and unhelpful thoughts.

4. *Fatigue*: When we're tired, sick or run-down, or experiencing low mood and vitality, we are more likely to see problems, threats, and difficulties and to catastrophise.

It is useful to reflect on our own patterns, identify our own common triggers and examine how we can minimise them.

The most common cognitive distortion we fall into is thinking that events determine how we feel and what we do. Albert Ellis, an American psychologist, developed the ABC model to teach people that rather than events and circumstances, it is their thoughts and beliefs that cause their emotional and behavioural responses. The reason this is such an important distinction to make is because we can't always control what happens to us, but we can always control our interpretations and thoughts around our experiences.

Viktor Frankl, an Austrian psychologist and Holocaust survivor, wrote in his book *Man's Search for Meaning* how the Nazis could, and did, take everything from him; his possessions, his family, and his freedom; but the one thing they could never take was his ability to choose his response. *'Between stimulus and response there is a gap, and within that gap lies our power to choose. Within that gap lies our human freedom.'*

This is mental agility, having the ability to look at circumstances from multiple perspectives.

Thinking traps get in the way of this mental agility.

This is how we think it works

A – Activating Event

(Negative Event or Circumstance)

↘

C - Consequence

(Feelings/Behaviors)

This is how it actually works
ABC Cognitive Model

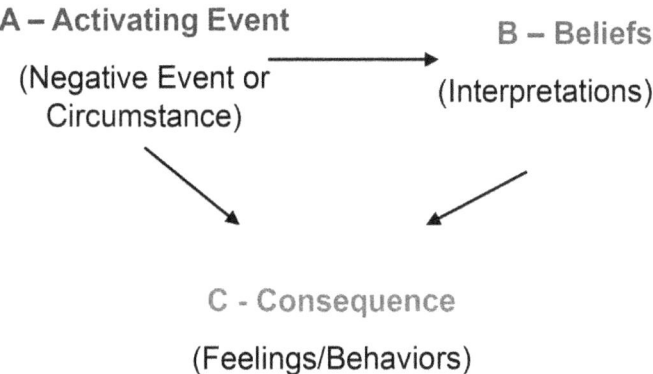

In Albert Ellis's ABC model, the A represents the activating event, the thing that happens. The B represents our beliefs about the event, essentially what we are saying to ourselves. The C represents the consequences, which are our subsequent reactions and emotions.

Most people believe that the A, the activating event, determines the C, the consequences. For example, I get fired from my ideal job, and as a consequence I am devastated and unable to function for weeks. In reality there is an in-between step, the B; what we believe, what we say to ourselves, what meaning we ascribe to the event. So if my belief is *Maybe I wasn't good enough for this job to begin with; I'll never find a job like this again*, then yes, I will be devastated. However, if my belief is *They have no right to fire me. I didn't do anything wrong. There are so many people less competent than me in this company*, then the consequence will be anger and rage. And if my belief is *I'll find another job. This job helped me see that it's possible to do work I love and get paid for it*, the consequence might be that I feel a little sad, but I'm mainly okay. In all three cases, the activating event is the same, but the consequences differ because of my beliefs and thoughts about the event. Thinking traps get in the way of our having this mental agility to see circumstances from different perspectives.

There are a number of common thinking traps we fall into. Some of the most common are:

1. *Mind Reading.* This is when we assume we know what others are thinking or, alternatively, we expect others to know what we're thinking. Example: *My manager didn't smile at me this morning; he must be mad at me.*

2. *Fortune Telling.* This is when we assume the worst and act as if it's a fact. Example: *I'm not going to go for the promotion because I probably won't get the position anyway.*

3. *Me Trap.* This is when we believe we are the cause of every setback or problem, even when events aren't under our control. Example: *My date is quiet; that must mean he'd prefer to be with someone else.*

4. *Them Trap.* This is when we believe that others are the sole cause of our problems and setbacks. Example: *My team has missed its target this month; they just aren't motivated and don't care about their work.*

5. *Disqualifying the Positive.* This is when we dismiss a positive experience by downplaying it's importance. Example: *My friend just gave me a compliment; I wonder what they want from me.*

6. *Labelling.* This is when we assign ourselves a negative label. Example: *I can't believe I made a mistake filling out that form and they had to return it to me. I'm such a loser. I'm a failure. What an idiot.*

7. *Black-and-White Thinking.* This is when we use words such as every, always, and never. Things are either good or bad, a success or failure, with nothing in between. In reality, nothing in life is absolute and things exist in various shades of grey. Example: *Most people say they really enjoyed my presentation, but one person said they couldn't hear me very well, and it's all I can think about.*

It can be very useful to ask which trap you most commonly fall into, to identify your own patterns, and also to consider the circumstances or events that encourage you to become entrapped. In many cases we find we are more prone to unhelpful thinking patterns when we are depleted in some way; stressed, anxious, worried, overworked, not getting enough sleep, not exercising, or eating a nutrient-poor diet.

The first step in negating unhelpful thinking patterns is building self-awareness around our thinking. Mindfulness and present-moment awareness are helpful for this. The next step involves identifying the unhelpful thought or belief; then we can look for evidence as to its accuracy or inaccuracy and finally formulate a more helpful and empowering new thought or belief that will help us more effectively engage with life. This is termed real-time resilience.

As an example, imagine giving a presentation at work to secure a new contract. Suppose the presentation doesn't go so well and you think *I'm just not good enough*. Firstly, you might look for evidence that supports this assumption. You might think:

- *I made a mess of this project*
- *The result is less than I had hoped*
- *At times my communication was poor and ineffective*
- *Ultimately, we didn't get the contract*

Next, you would look for evidence against the assumption:

- *I am one of the top three salespeople in the company*
- *My presentation was successful last time*
- *People are always telling me how much they enjoy my presentations*
- *This time I just didn't have time to prepare*

Essentially, we are using data to prove to ourselves why our thought isn't true. The final step is coming up with a more empowering thought, such as *I am more than good enough, but I'm just not feeling it lately because I had a few things in a row that didn't go according to plan.*

Sentence Starters

Sentence starters are a useful way of doing this in real time as the unhelpful thoughts arise. Sentence starters are just phrases that we have to hand that we can call on when the need arises. There are three useful ones that cover most situations.

1. *That's Not True Because* . . . can be used when we want to provide evidence that a particular thought or belief isn't true. For example, if we have the thought *I'm so useless at my job*, we can counter that thought with the statement *That's not true because I won lots of new clients last quarter* or *That's not true because I often receive positive feedback from customers.*

2. *Another Way Of Looking At This Is* . . . can be used when we want to reframe a way we perceive a situation. For example, if we have the thought *I'm always messing things up; I'm just no good at this*, we can counter that thought with the statement *A more helpful way to see this is that although I didn't do great on this occasion, I know I can do better next time.*

3. *If X Happens, I Will Y . . .* can be used when we want to create a contingency plan and is especially useful for catastrophic thinking. For example, before giving a presentation, you may begin to get nervous and become worried that your mind will go blank and you'll make a fool of yourself. In this situation, you might create a plan by saying *If I get nervous, I will take three long, slow, deep breaths to calm myself down and have my notes to hand in case I need to refer to them.*

When a counterproductive thought pops into our head, we can use these sentence starters to access a more helpful thought or belief. This technique often reminds me of the Whac-a-Mole casino game where we whack the moles with a mallet every time they raise their heads! In a similar way when an unhelpful thought arises, we immediately replace it with an empowering one.

Catastrophising

Catastrophising is one of the most debilitating thinking traps we can fall into and can often lead to the experience of overwhelming anxiety. For example, we may miss an important deadline at work and begin to spiral into thoughts such as:

Oh no, my manager will give me a poor review, leading to I'll lose my job, then

I won't be able to pay the mortgage, and on to
I won't be able to afford to send my kids to college.
When we catastrophise, thoughts build one on top of the other, making each a little worse than the one before it. This results in our irrational worries feeling more rational and believable than they actually are. Each concern is replaced by one that's a little bit worse, and so our worries appear real. Often it takes the perspective of someone else for us to realise our thoughts are unrealistic. In general, there are three types of catastrophising:

1. *Downward Spiral.* This is when each successive thought we have becomes progressively worse, leading to a worst-case scenario. For example, perhaps we're working on a busy project and our boss calls to say the three-week deadline has been brought forward to the end of this week. Our thoughts spiral from *There's no way I can get this done* to *The boss is going to be so mad* to *I'll never get that promotion* to *I'll lose my job, and that's the last three years of my career gone down the drain* to *My career is ruined.*

2. *Scattershot Thinking.* This is when one negative thought leads to thoughts of many discrete, different, bad outcomes. As in the above example with the shortened project deadline, we might think *There's no way I can get that done*, but then we might jump to *I was going to take a couple days' holidays, and there's no way I can do that now* and then to *I won't be able to bring my*

wife for a meal tonight as planned and then to *I won't have time to exercise this week.*

3. *Circling.* This is when our negative thoughts have one primary theme and we keep going round and round with different variations of the same thought. As in the example above, we might think *I'll never have enough time* along with several variations, such as *How am I supposed to get this done by the end of the week?* and *There is so much work to do; I'll never have enough time* and *There are only twenty-four hours in the day.*

So what can we do about catastrophic thinking? A useful technique for breaking the cycle is called Worst Case, Best Case, Most Likely Scenario. It involves dividing a page into three columns and naming the left *Worst Case*, the right *Best Case*, and the centre *Most Likely*.

First, we go through the worst case, which is what would happen if everything went completely pear shaped. Then we go through the best case; what it would look like if things went so well, they exceeded our wildest dreams. Neither of these has to be realistic; in fact, the more we exaggerate them, the better. This then gives us guide rails; we know that things probably won't go as bad as the absolute worst case, nor are they likely to go as well as the ultimate best case. Then we go to the centre column and fill in what the most probable or most likely outcome will be. Now we have limits to work within so we can focus on a plan. It's helpful to put all this down on paper, at least until we're familiar with the technique, rather than attempting to go through this in our head.

Your boss asks you to give a presentation to a group of potential investors.		
Worst Case Thoughts	**Most Likely Thoughts**	**Best Case Thoughts**
I'm going to make a fool of myself	It will take me a long time to prep	Without any prep, I'll be amazing
My boss will be furious	I'll be really nervous	My boss will promote me
I'll get fired	I'll do my best	I'll become CEO
I won't be able to find a new job	It will go okay	Because I'm so good at presenting I'll quit and become a speaker!
I won't be able to pay my bills.	I'll get feedback and improve	I'm famous
I'll go bankrupt	If asked to do it again I'll be better next time	I'll get on Oprah
I'll lose my house		My boss trusts me
I'll be all alone		No need to work!

Story: The Glass of Water

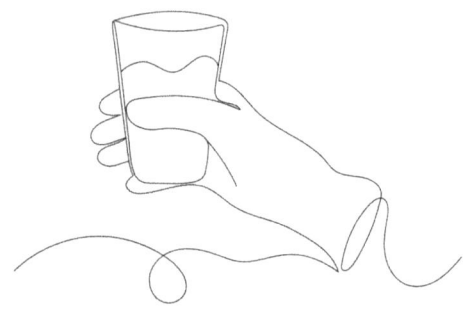

During a lecture, a professor of psychology held up a glass half full of water. All the students were expecting the often-asked question *'Is the glass half full or is the glass half empty?'* But instead, the professor surprised them all by asking, *'How heavy is this glass of water I'm holding?'*

Students shouted out various guesses and answers as to the weight of the glass of water.

The professor responded, *'The absolute weight of the glass doesn't matter. It all depends on how long I hold it. If I hold it for a minute or two, it's fairly light. If I hold it for an hour, its weight might make my arm ache. If I hold it for a day, my arm will likely cramp up and feel completely numb, forcing me to drop the glass on the floor. In each case, the weight of the glass doesn't change, but the longer I hold it, the heavier it feels.'*

'Your thoughts, anxieties, and worries in life are very much like this glass of water. Think about them for a short time, and there's no problem. However, think of them for a longer period, and you may begin to feel uncomfortable. Think of them for a period of days or weeks and you will feel completely numb, paralysed, and ineffective, incapable of taking action.

'What happens when we add more water?' he asked the class. *'What if you fill the glass to the top? Never forget,'* he explained, *'the secret is always to just put the glass down.'*

In life, always remember that we need to let go of our negative thoughts, anxieties, and worries. Ruminating about them, although we may feel like we are problem-solving, just leads to paralysis. Rather than this paralysis, choose more empowering thoughts and take action. Emotionally intelligent people put the glass down and figure out a better strategy.

CHAPTER 8

The Power of Positive Emotions

Tool: Gratitude
Pillar: Positive Emotions

> *If the only prayer you say in your life is
> 'Thank you', that would suffice.*
>
> —Meister Eckhart

Staying with the P in the REVAMP model, the practice of gratitude stands out as one of the most researched and impactful wellbeing interventions. By cultivating gratitude, we can actively increase the presence of positive emotions in our lives, which significantly enhances our overall wellbeing. Positive emotions such as excitement, enthusiasm, love, joy, awe, interest, and pride enrich our life experience. It makes sense that if we consciously create more moments of joy or experience deeper feelings of love throughout our day, we elevate our sense of wellbeing and bring greater meaning and fulfilment to our lives.

Exercise

Gently close your eyes. Bring yourself into the present by taking three long, slow, deep breaths. Imagine you're feeling stressed. You are anxious, worried, irritable, and overwhelmed. Where do you feel that in your body? Tension in your neck, shoulders, forehead? Jaw clenched, breathing shallow? That familiar feeling in the pit of your stomach?

Imagine that you've finished your day's work. You arrive home and open the door to your kitchen. Inside is your partner, kids, or housemates. Play through the scenario in your head. Remember you are stressed, worried, anxious, overwhelmed.

> What thoughts are you going to have?
> What is your focus going to be?
> How will your conversations go?
> What decisions will you make?
> What are your interactions like?
> What kind of energy do you bring to the situation?
> And as a result, what sort of experience will you have?

Okay, open your eyes and shake it off. Shake your wrists, your fingers, your arms, your elbows, shoulders up to your ears. Make circles with your shoulders and then move your head in a circular motion three times clockwise and three times anticlockwise.

Close your eyes again. Take three nice, slow, deep breaths.

This time I want you to imagine the exact opposite scenario.

This time you are enthusiastic, inspired, full of fun. You feel loving, caring, light.

Where do you feel this in your body? What is the expression in your eyes, your smile? Your jaw is nice and relaxed, shoulders loose, freedom in your body.

Once again you arrive home and open the door to your kitchen. Inside is your partner, kids, or housemates. As you enter, they can see straight away that you are in a positive state. In this scenario:

>What thoughts are you going to have?
>What is your focus going to be?
>How will your conversations go?
>What decisions will you make?
>What are your interactions like?
>What kind of energy do you bring to the situation?

And as a result, what sort of experience will you have?

Our emotional state has a profound effect on our bodies. It alters our brain chemistry, our neurotransmitters, our hormones, and which neural pathways are active. This has knock-on effects on our thoughts, which determine our actions and therefore our results and experiences.

It's as if two different versions of us walk into that kitchen and as a result, we have different thoughts, take different actions, and have wildly different results and experiences. Therefore, we can't discount the role that our emotions play in our day-to-day lives and in the results and experiences we have.

Across is a chart listing common emotions, both positive and negative. Look through the list and place a tick beside those emotions you have experienced in the last week. Have you experienced joy, pride, serenity, love, inspiration, interest, or gratitude? On the negative side, have you felt stress, fear, guilt, sadness, hate, anxiety, anger, shame, distrust, or overwhelm?

Positive	Negative
☐ Joy	☐ Stress
☐ Pride	☐ Fear
☐ Serenity	☐ Guilt
☐ Love	☐ Sadness
☐ Inspiration	☐ Hate
☐ Interest	☐ Anxiety
☐ Awe	☐ Anger
☐ Gratitude	☐ Shame
☐ Hope	☐ Distrust
☐ Amusement	☐ Overwhelm
% Recently _____	% Recently _____

Have you ever stopped to reflect on the emotions you've experienced? Think about what triggered them. What were the circumstances? Who were you with? Were you at home or work? Exploring these questions can help you understand your emotions better, revealing patterns and trends. This practice is a simple yet powerful way to increase self-awareness. Often, we go through life experiencing emotions without really noticing them. They can linger for days, weeks, or even months, while we remain unaware. Pausing to reflect is the first step to understanding. Once we gain that awareness, the next step is learning how to adapt and move on from emotions that no longer serve us.

Chosing Our Emotional State

Many of us feel trapped by our emotions, believing we have no control over them. But the truth is much more empowering. We can choose our emotional state. This isn't about chasing perpetual happiness or forcing ourselves into unrealistic positivity. Instead, it's about recognising that emotions are valuable signals. Our emotions respond to our environment, and while we might label some as 'positive' and others as 'negative,' they all play important roles.

Think about a time when you felt fear. That fear likely prompted action that protected you or your loved ones. While fear might be labelled as negative, its outcome was positive. The goal isn't to avoid so-called negative emotions but to allow ourselves to fully experience the rich spectrum of human feelings. This permission to be human means acknowledging both joys and challenges without getting stuck in any one emotion. No emotion is inherently problematic, but issues arise when we dwell on them for too long. If we remain emotionally unaware, certain emotions can persist unnecessarily. For instance, feeling sad is a normal part of life, but when sadness becomes prolonged, it can evolve into depression, which is a more serious concern. Similarly, occasional worry is natural, but when worry becomes a constant state, it turns into anxiety.

The key is to understand our emotions, appreciate their significance, and learn when and how to let them go. By doing so, we cultivate emotional agility and create a more balanced, fulfilling experience of life.

Emotion is not the issue; rather, the issue is the length of time we stay in that emotion.

Next it's helpful to consider, why do we have emotions anyway? What purpose do they serve? What advantage have they provided to humankind? From an evolutionary point of view, negative emotions enabled our ancestors to survive. Negative emotions are all about survival and stimulate our stress response or fight-or-flight response. When we are in a negative state, our focus narrows. Our only concern is *How can I protect myself? How can I escape this danger? How can I survive this crisis?* So we have this narrow focus in which we are concerned only with ourselves, giving us tunnel vision and limiting our choices.

All negative emotions have specific actions associated with them. For example, if you feel anger, you are always going to want to respond by doing just one thing and one thing alone, and that is to fight back. In a similar way, feeling fear is always going to compel you to run away. Shame will always make you want to hide, and guilt will always make you want to respond by making amends. As a result, we are very limited in the actions we take when we experience negative emotions.

Up until the late 1990s, nothing much was known about positive emotions apart from the fact that it felt good to feel them. Barbara Fredrickson, an American professor in the department of psychology at the University of North Carolina, wrote a paper titled '*What Good Are Positive Emotions?*' She realised that positive emotions[10] had to serve some purpose other than merely feeling good and began to investigate the evolutionary advantage of them. She discovered that their main purpose was to help our ancestors build resources, either personal or collective, a theory she called Broaden-and-Build.

We feel positive emotions only when we have a sense of safety and security and we're not under threat. Under these circumstances, positive emotions allow us to build resources so that instead of having a narrow focus on ourselves, we begin to think globally, of the '*we*' rather than the '*me*'. We are much more likely to be cooperative with other people, to collaborate with others, and to be creative. Instead of our focus being internal; *my problems, my issues, my difficulties*; we are more outward looking. We want to interact with people, to engage with the world and the environment around us.

Consider what happens when we are in a low mood. Our head is down, we are preoccupied, we don't want to interact with people or to engage with others. In contrast to this, when we are positive and upbeat, our head is up, we make eye contact, we interact, we engage, we chat, and we are much more open and receptive. This is Barbara Fredrickson's *Broaden-and-Build* theory in action.

In fact, when we are positive, not only are we psychologically and emotionally more available and open to the world around us, but studies have also revealed that we have a physiological response that makes our environment more visible to us. In a positive emotional state, our peripheral vision increases by about 25% so that we are more outward looking and more aware of our environment and surroundings.

Why is it important to prioritise positive emotions when we experience both positive and negative ones? You might think that life naturally balances out – getting out on the right side of the bed one day and the wrong side the next. However, it's not that straightforward. Our brains are wired with a negativity bias, meaning we naturally focus more on threats, problems, and what's going wrong in our lives.

Think of it this way: our brains are like Velcro for the bad and Teflon for the good.[11] Negative experiences stick with us, demanding our attention and causing us to dwell on them, making them harder to shake off. On the flip side, positive experiences tend to slide away unnoticed, or if we do see them, we quickly forget or dismiss them. While good things happen around us every day, our natural tendency is to overlook and undervalue them.

From an evolutionary standpoint, our negativity bias played a crucial role in our survival as a species. Picture your prehistoric ancestors navigating ancient forests or open plains. Paying attention to threats, like a poisonous snake at their feet, was far more important than spotting opportunities, such as a ripe apple on a branch. Missing the snake could mean death, while missing the apple simply meant going hungry. While our negativity bias was vital for survival in the past, it holds far less relevance in today's modern world.

Given its lasting influence, prioritising positivity in our lives has become essential for enhancing wellbeing. Now, imagine this. Today, I'm expecting the delivery of an extraordinary medicine to the pharmacy. It's brand new, straight off the production line. Because you're reading this, I'm offering it to you completely free for life. It comes with zero side effects, and the level of research behind it is undeniable and rigorous. You can trust that everything I'm about to share with you is accurate, unchanging, and completely reliable.If you take this medicine on a daily basis, it's going to benefit your:

- immune system, helping you fight off colds and flus more effectively
- sleep quality, making you sleep deeper and more soundly
- life satisfaction and contentedness

- vitality, giving you more energy to go about your daily business
- optimism, such that you will look to the future with a greater sense of hope
- social orientation, so that you will find it easier to relate to people and get on better with them

Absolutely fantastic! That's an impressive list! Okay, hands up; who wants some? No catches; there are zero catches. But even better, there's more:

This medicine can do extraordinary things for your health, like:

- Reduces cortisol, the stress hormone, promoting better overall health.
- Lowers inflammatory biomarkers, tackling inflammation that contributes to many diseases.
- Helps decrease blood pressure and cut cholesterol levels, benefiting cardiovascular health.
- Improves mindset by reducing self-absorption and materialistic tendencies.
- Delivers profound and immediate improvements to your sense of wellbeing.

Surely, this would be hailed as the next multibillion-dollar blockbuster, right? But here's the twist. This medicine already exists, and you already have access to it. *It's called gratitude.*

Gratitude is the most extensively researched intervention in positive psychology, with an evidence base that is rock solid. At its core, gratitude is a sense of thankfulness or a feeling of joy and appreciation for good fortune or kindness received. Remarkably, practising gratitude can deliver profound and immediate improvements to your sense of wellbeing, requiring less time than brushing your teeth each day. It's breathtakingly simple, and sometimes, the simplest practices are the most powerful.

What is important here is the word *practice*. We need to actively create moments to feel gratitude, rather than simply knowing that it's beneficial. Truly experiencing the positive emotions of gratitude is what transforms its impact. When it comes to the benefits for our body and mind, it's not about checking off a list of things we're grateful for; it's about immersing ourselves in the feelings of appreciation. By choosing to focus on things that bring us gratitude, we can give our wellbeing a much-needed uplift.

While the world is undeniably filled with challenges such as tragedy, conflict, illness, and hardship; our natural negativity bias ensures we won't overlook those realities. Gratitude, instead, offers a gentle shift in perspective. It reminds us of the magic, beauty, and wonder that also exist in abundance. The very fact that you are alive is miraculous. Think about the incredible processes occurring within your body every second, such as the ability to breathe, see, hear, move, and experience the world through your senses. Reflect on your heart, lungs, muscles, and bones, all working tirelessly to support you as you explore this awe-inspiring planet. Gratitude helps us attune to life's extraordinary wonders, grounding us in positivity and possibility.

The true wonder lies in how easily we take it all for granted. Often, we fail to fully appreciate the world around us, barely bringing its marvels into our awareness or consciousness. Consider this an invitation to wear your 'gratitude goggles' at least once a day. By shifting the lens through which you view the world, you can uncover the beauty and abundance that surround you.

The Power of Gratitude

Positive psychology teaches us that its interventions truly work when we take the time to apply them. Gratitude, in particular, stands out as one of the most powerful tools in this practice. But what makes gratitude so impactful?

1. **Pressing Pause on Life.** Gratitude gives us the chance to pause amidst the chaos of our bustling lives. Modern life often feels like a relentless race as we juggle work, family, health, finances, and more, all while chasing a bigger, better version of what we already have. We hurriedly move forward, rarely stopping to appreciate the present moment. However, when crisis strikes, what do most people

wish for? They often say, 'I just want things to go back to normal.' It's a telling reminder. The simple 'normal' that we once overlooked can actually be extraordinary. Gratitude invites us to cherish both the remarkable and the seemingly routine moments. It's through gratitude that we find beauty in our everyday lives, often hidden in plain sight.

2. **Broadening our Perspective.** Developing a regular gratitude practice allows us to lower our gratitude threshold. Consider this staggering reality: over one billion people lack access to clean drinking water, and around eight hundred million people go to bed every night with an empty stomach. For these individuals, many of the things we take for granted would be seen as extraordinary blessings. A secure roof over our heads, clean air, electricity, the internet, or simply a smartphone. These aren't universal experiences, yet they are integral parts of our lives. Now pause and ask yourself this question. If someone lacking these privileges would feel overwhelmed with gratitude for what you have right now, why aren't we feeling the same way? Gratitude opens our eyes to the abundance in even the smallest aspects of our lives and nudges us to live with deeper appreciation.

Now if they would be so grateful for these things, that leaves the question: Why aren't we?

The reason for this is a phenomenon known as *adaptation*. It is our capacity to adjust to adversity; be it natural disasters, social upheaval, or personal struggles that has contributed significantly to our survival and progression as a species. However, this same ability to adapt can work against us when it comes to recognising and appreciating the positives in our lives. Over time, the initial joy or excitement brought on by new experiences or accomplishments fades into normalcy. For example, that new car we bought and would look at admiringly every time we sat in it no longer thrills us in the same way. That girlfriend or boyfriend we couldn't bear to be apart from for five minutes has now become our husband or wife that we wake up beside every morning, yet we barely look over to their side of the bed when we awaken.

This is why nurturing a habit of gratitude is so essential. By consciously acknowledging the blessings in our lives, we counteract this natural tendency to take them for granted, ensuring that joy and appreciation remain at the forefront of our daily experiences.

3. **Gratitude is a Prosocial Emotion.** It fosters meaningful connections with others, which are integral to enhancing wellbeing. Psychologist Sarah Igoe developed the '*Find, Bind, and Remind*' theory[12] of gratitude, which highlights how expressing gratitude helps in three key ways. Firstly, it allows us to find new friendships by creating positive interactions. Secondly,

it strengthens and binds existing relationships by deepening emotional bonds. Lastly, it reminds us of those who have supported us in the past, encouraging recognition of their role in shaping who we are today.

4. **Gratitude makes us less Materialistic.** At its core, gratitude is about appreciating and wanting what we already have. This mindset reduces the desire for material possessions such as the latest gadgets or luxury items, which are often pursued in the belief that they will bring happiness. By focusing on what is already present in our lives, we find contentment and alleviate the constant urge for newer, bigger, or better things.

5. **Gratitude reduces Social Comparison.** Comparing ourselves to others is a significant detriment to our wellbeing. No matter our achievements or possessions, there will always be someone who seems to have more or be better in some way. Gratitude, however, shifts the focus inwards, allowing us to value and cherish what we have rather than fixating on what others possess. By doing so, it diminishes the tendency to make unfavourable comparisons, fostering a healthier self-perception.

6. **Gratitude counters our Negativity Bias.** Humans have a natural inclination to focus on potential threats and challenges; a negativity bias that can

overshadow the positives in life. Gratitude acts as a powerful antidote, training the mind to notice and savour the good. It shifts attention away from the problems and towards the blessings, helping us acknowledge and find joy in the often-overlooked aspects of our everyday lives.

7. **Gratitude is most effective when it's both Reflective and Expressive.** Reflecting on gratitude involves taking a moment each day to pause and consider or write down the things you appreciate in your life. This practice helps to cultivate mindfulness and reinforces positivity by focusing on what truly matters. Meanwhile, expressing gratitude brings it to life by actively thanking the people around you for their contributions, no matter how small they may seem. Whether it's someone holding the door open, offering a kind word, or lending a helping hand, acknowledging these gestures can foster stronger connections and promote a sense of goodwill. Gratitude thrives in action as much as in thought, making it a powerful tool for enhancing both personal and social wellbeing. There's a lovely saying:

Feeling gratitude and not expressing it is like wrapping a present and not giving it.

—William Arthur Ward

So how do we go about practicing gratitude in our lives? One way is to keep a gratitude journal where you write down a couple of things you are grateful for on a daily basis. It is helpful to place this in a visible location to remind you to engage with the practice; for example, on your bedside locker as opposed to in it!

A more useful variation of this is the *Three Good Things* exercise.

Three Good Things

Another effective way to cultivate gratitude is through the '*Three Good Things*' practice. Unlike a traditional gratitude journal, which can often become repetitive and lose its impact over time, this approach encourages us to identify three positive events from the past twenty-four hours and reflect on how we contributed to them. This deliberate process not only ensures variety but also prompts us to actively search for meaningful and positive moments in our daily lives. By doing so, the practice maintains its freshness and effectiveness, allowing us to develop a deeper appreciation for the small but significant joys that each day brings.Let's give the last word to a very wise man indeed:

> *There are two ways to live your life. One is as though nothing is a miracle. The other is as though everything is a miracle.*
>
> —Albert Einstein

Story: Happiness Is Within You

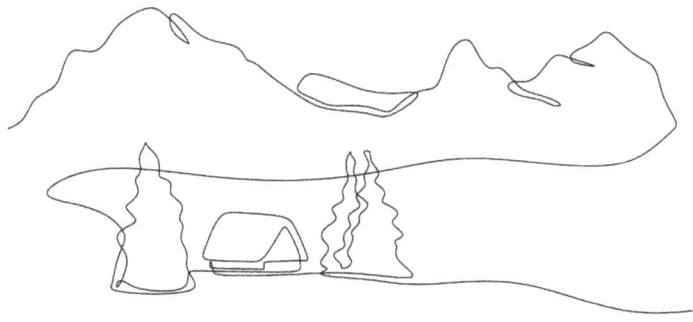

Once there was a very successful businessman who was always worried and restless. He heard of a wise guru who lived on top of a nearby mountain and held the secret to everlasting peace and happiness, so he decided to pay him a visit. He climbed the mountain, passing over rivers and streams, over rocks and boulders, until eventually he reached the top of the mountain. When he met the guru, he said, *'I believe you have the secret to lasting peace and happiness. Can you share it with me?'*

The guru replied, *'Of course, but you must return early tomorrow morning, and then we will talk.'*

Feeling satisfied and excited, the businessman returned back down the mountain. Early the following morning he set off again up the mountain. As before, he passed over rivers and streams, over rocks and boulders, until eventually he reached the top of the mountain. When he came to the hut where the guru lived, he found him on his hands and knees outside the hut, intently looking for something. It was clear the guru had lost something, so the businessman asked if he could assist him.

'*Please,*' said the guru, '*I have lost my most precious and holy necklace that I have worn since I was a young man and can't find it anywhere.*'

The businessman got down on his hands and knees and helped in the search. Twenty minutes passed, then forty, then sixty, and eventually the businessman, tiring of the search, said, '*Where were you when you lost the necklace? Do you remember?*'

'*Oh yes,*' said the guru. '*I was inside my hut!*'

'*If your necklace fell inside the hut, then why are you looking out here?*' replied the businessman in annoyance. '*How will you find the thing here outside which is inside there?*'

The guru looked up at the businessman and gently smiled. '*That, my dear man, is the solution to your problem. Happiness and lasting peace are inside you, but you continue to look for them outside in the external world. The entire world searches outside themselves for the happiness and peace that have been inside all along.*'

In life, inner peace and happiness are within everyone but get covered by layers of conditioning, social hypnosis, and misguided expectations. We tend to chase happiness through career, wealth, money, and success, only to find that chasing these things is a never-ending treadmill.

> *Happiness and peace are two basic characteristics of every human that do not need to be chased; they just need to be revealed.*

CHAPTER 9

Creating Change

Tool: Habit Formation
Pillar: REVAMP

*Small steps in the right direction can
be the biggest steps of your life.*

—Naeem Callaway

Knowledge vs Applied Knowledge

The preceding eight chapters detail science-backed, research-based tools and techniques that are proven to boost wellbeing. However, they come with a caveat: We have to do the work! Often in life we suffer from what is called the knowledge fallacy. This is a belief that just because we know something, we are halfway there. Unfortunately, however, unlike what we are led to believe with the saying *Knowledge is power*, it is more accurate and correct to say *Knowledge is power . . . but only if we use it!*

The distinction between '*knowledge*' and '*applied knowledge*' is an important one to understand. As an illustration, imagine if I were the world's leading authority on strength and conditioning. I knew all there was to know about nutrition, exercise, sets, repetitions, creatine, branch chain amino acids, and protein intake. However, if I never set foot in a gym, lifted a dumbbell, or curled a bicep, that information would be useless and I would see no alteration in my body definition. It's all down to taking regular, consistent action.

Chris Peterson, one of the founding fathers of positive psychology, put it well when he said, '*When we know what we know, why do we continue to do what we do?*' Knowledge is only the first step, and more often than not the lack of it isn't the stumbling block to change. Which of us doesn't actually know what to do when it comes to losing weight, for example? The knowledge may be there, but change can be difficult as we continuously fall back into old habits.

Key to change is starting small. In fact, the smaller the better. Often we are tempted to change everything overnight, only to find after a couple of days that we have created a situation that is just not sustainable. Small changes that are easy to apply are also easier to repeat, and repetition is key to change. We have already discussed how '*Nerves that fire together, wire together*' and the concept of neuroplasticity. Just like when a skier skis down a snow covered mountain creating tracks in the snow, repetition deepens the groove so that it can be difficult to redirect ourselves. We have been doing things one way for so long that it can feel uncomfortable to deviate. However, despite the common belief that we can't teach an old dog new tricks, in reality, it is never too late to change.

Key to this process is creating small, repeatable habits. Too often we rely on motivation alone. However, motivation is a finite resource and often lets us down when we are in some way depleted: tired, hungry, or stressed.

The Habit Loop

Research shows that 40% of the actions we take on a daily basis are governed by habit, not actual decisions, meaning much of what we do is not our conscious choice but happens because we did it yesterday, and the day before, and the day before that again. We always fold our arms in the same way, put our legs into our jeans in the same sequence, and repeat many of our daily tasks in a very predictable manner. Habits are useful, as they allow us to free up mental energy, and to a certain extent they allow us to dispense with the need for self-regulation. As a result, we never have to motivate ourselves every morning to brush our teeth! It's an ingrained habit, a done deal, without any conscious input from us. This is where we want to get to when it comes to forming our new wellbeing habits.

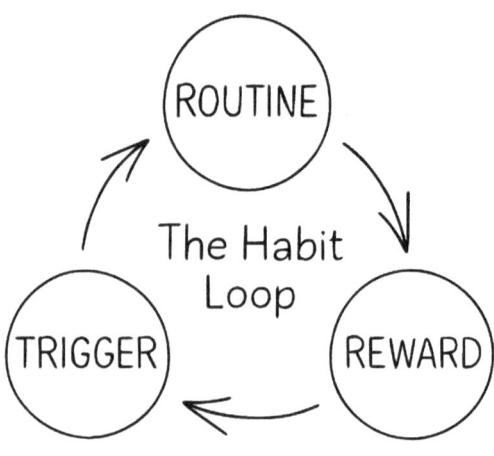

All habits follow what is called a neurological habit loop consisting of three elements: a trigger, a routine, and a reward. Here is an example of this loop: We enter the kitchen in the morning and see the kettle (trigger). We boil the kettle and make a cup of coffee (routine). We experience the caffeine, the warmth, and aroma of the coffee (reward). All three elements must be present, with the reward resulting in a boost of dopamine in our brains, reinforcing the habit, and as a consequence making it hard to break a habit. A process called habit stacking is a convenient and effective way to instil new habits into our day as we anchor a new routine to an existing habit loop.

Example would be *After I pour my coffee in the morning, I will meditate for two minutes* or *After I brush my teeth at night, I will complete my Three Good Things gratitude exercise.* We keep the same trigger and reward and simply stack an additional habit on top. In fact, this is the whole basis for the use of nicotine replacement therapy in smokers who wish to quit. A smoker gets a craving for a cigarette (trigger), they alter the routine from cigarette to nicotine gum (routine), and they retain the experience of the jolt of nicotine (reward).

Another way to increase our chance of success when it comes to instilling new wellbeing habits is to use two of the strongest cues when it comes to forming and maintaining habits; namely, environment and time. In a study by Professor Peter Gollwitzer at New York University, students were given a cue by the professor,[13] which was an assignment on how they spent their winter break. He divided the students into two groups. One was told they had to submit the assignment by December 27, while the second group was given the same date but had to tell the professor when and where they would be when they completed it. Remarkably, only 32% of the first group, compared to 71% of the second group, submitted the assignment on time. The professor had used two of the most common cues to trigger a habit: time and location. This experiment has been replicated with similar results across a wide range of scenarios.

In a related study of 250 subjects in the UK aimed at supporting people in establishing an exercise habit, participants were divided into three groups. One tracked how often they exercised, the second were also given a motivational talk on the benefits of exercise, and the third were also asked to formulate a plan for their exercise by completing the sentence '*During the next week I will complete 20 minutes of exercise on (DAY) at (TIME) in (PLACE).*' Of the first group, 35%, 38% of the second group, and 91% of the third group successfully completed the required exercise. This is called creating an implementation intention and is a useful tool when making change to our routines.

Story: The Starfish Story

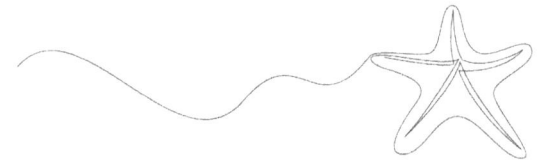

One day an old man was walking along a beautiful, isolated beach. He came to a stretch on which thousands and thousands of starfish had washed up, as far as the eye could see, stretching in both directions.

In the distance he could see a little girl approaching, who paused and bent down every so often.

'May I ask what it is that you are doing?' he said as she neared him.

'I'm throwing the starfish back into the sea. They can't return to the sea by themselves, and they will die unless I throw them back into the water.'

'But there are miles and miles of beach, and there are thousands upon thousands of starfish. You won't really be able to make much of a difference!'

The little girl bent down, picked up a starfish, and looked the man in the eye as she threw the starfish back into the water. *'I sure made a difference to that one, mister!'* she exclaimed.

Often we can become paralysed by the enormity of a task, feel that all is hopeless and that we can never make a difference or make progress. However, each journey begins with a small step, and every step we take brings us that little bit closer to our destination.

Bonus Chapter

By starting small, staying consistent, and leaning on the REVAMP framework, you can begin to improve your wellbeing one day at a time. Remember, even the smallest step forward is progress!

Here are some key takeaways to remember, followed by simple, practical action steps to take to successfully integrate REVAMP into your life.

Key Takeaways

Knowledge vs. Action

- Knowing something isn't enough. Real change requires consistent, practical application of knowledge.
- Small, consistent steps are more impactful and sustainable than trying to change everything at once.

The Power of Habits

- Around 40% of actions are governed by habits, which free up mental energy for other tasks.

- Habits revolve around a loop of trigger, routine, reward and can be adjusted using habit-stacking techniques or external cues like time and location.

The Importance of Starting Small
- Small, repeatable habits are easier to maintain and build long-term momentum.
- Motivation is finite, but habits, once formed, become automatic.

The Role of Environment and Timing
- Structuring your environment and establishing specific time-based routines significantly increases habit success rates.
- Studies highlight the importance of planning actions, using cues like when and where, to achieve goals effectively.

Mindset Shifts

- Neuroplasticity means it's never too late to adopt new habits or change old patterns.
- Progress, not perfection, is key. Every small step counts towards overall transformation.

The WellBeing Revamp Framework (REVAMP)

- Relationships boost wellbeing and should be consistently nurtured and prioritised.
- Engagement involves being present in the moment to enhance experiences and flow states.
- Vitality is influenced by proper diet, sufficient movement, and quality sleep.
- Achievement requires setting meaningful and motivating goals for balance across life areas.
- Meaning provides purpose and fulfilment, which can be found in everyday actions.
- Positive emotions shape our outlook and can be intentionally cultivated.

Action Items

Identify a Focus Area

Reflect on one area where you'd like to improve (e.g., building better habits, enhancing relationships, or increasing vitality).

Implement Habit Stacking

Attach one new habit to an existing routine using the formula After I [current habit], I will [new habit]. Example: After brushing my teeth, I will note three things I'm grateful for.

Set an Implementation Intention

Plan your next action step using this framework: I will [action] on [day] at [time] in [location].

Optimise Your Environment

Modify your surroundings to encourage good habits and minimise distractions. For example, keep healthy snacks visible and easily accessible to support dietary goals.

Schedule Time for Reflection

Dedicate a few minutes daily to assess your progress and celebrate small wins. This reinforces positive behaviour and helps maintain motivation.

Address Negative Habits

Identify current negative habit loops and replace routines with healthier alternatives. For example, substitute evening scrolling on your phone with reading a book or a short walk.

Use External Cues

Set triggers like calendar reminders or morning routines to anchor positive actions and stay consistent.

Prioritise WellBeing Across All Areas

Balance all aspects of the REVAMP framework in your routine. Ensure your goals span relationships, vitality, meaning, and engagement for holistic wellbeing.

Take the Next Step Towards Transforming Your Wellbeing

So, you've made it to the end of *Your Wellbeing Revamp*, and I hope you're feeling inspired, a little clearer, and more in control of your own wellbeing.

If there's one thing I've learned through years of working in healthcare and wellbeing, it's this: small, intentional changes, performed consistently, can radically shift how we feel, think, and live. And now that you've taken the time to explore those changes through this book, you're already on the path.

Throughout my career as a community pharmacist, wellbeing educator, and founder of iThrive, I've seen the impact of daily habits on health and wellbeing, both positive and negative. That's exactly what pushed me to dive deeper into the science of wellbeing, studying stress management, yoga, clinical hypnosis, and applied positive psychology.

iThrive was born from a desire to help people just like you make real, lasting improvements to their wellbeing, without needing to turn their whole life upside down.

Whether it's through corporate workshops, group programmes, or one-on-one coaching my mission is simple: to help you feel good and function effectively using tools that are grounded in science and easy to put into practice.

You've done the reading. You've started reflecting. Maybe you've even begun experimenting with new habits. Now comes the exciting part, turning that insight into action.

So, what's next? If you'd like to continue this journey with more guidance and hands on support, I'd love to work with you. My flagship programmes, Your Wellbeing REVAMP, and The iThrive Wellbeing Experience, are designed to help you take what you've learned and integrate it into your everyday life.

Explore upcoming programmes by visiting iThrive.ie, or drop me a line at info@ithrive.ie. Type FREE GIFTS in the subject line and I'll forward you a copy of the key takeaways from the book plus a 21 Day Wellbeing Challenge to get you started.

Because your wellbeing isn't a luxury, it's your greatest asset. And it deserves your full attention and priority. Let's keep going, together!

References

[1] Killingsworth, M.A. & Gilbert, D.T., 2010. A wandering mind is an unhappy mind. *Science*, 330(6006), p.932. https://doi.org/10.1126/science.1192439

[2] Rill, P., 2014. *Triumphs of Experience: The Men of the Harvard Grant Study*. Activities, Adaptation & Aging, 38(4), pp.331–332. https://doi.org/10.1080/01924788.2014.966574

[3] Brown, E.G., Gallagher, S. & Creaven, A.M., 2018. Loneliness and acute stress reactivity: A systematic review of psychophysiological studies. *Psychophysiology*, 55(5), p.e13031. https://doi.org/10.1111/psyp.13031

[4] Li, H. & Xia, N., 2020. The role of oxidative stress in cardiovascular disease caused by social isolation and loneliness. *Redox Biology*, 37, p.101585. https://doi.org/10.1016/j.redox.2020.101585

[5] Fowler, J.H. & Christakis, N.A., 2008. Dynamic spread of happiness in a large social network: longitudinal analysis over 20 years in the Framingham Heart Study. *BMJ*, 337, a2338. https://doi.org/10.1136/bmj.a2338

[6] Lieberman, D.E., Pontzer, H., Cutright-Smith, E. & Raichlen, D.A., 2005. Why is the human gluteus so maximus? *American Journal of Physical Anthropology*. https://doi.org/10.1002/ajpa.20217

[7] Noetel, M. et al., 2024. Effect of exercise for depression: systematic review and network meta-analysis of randomised controlled trials. *BMJ*, 384, p.e075847. https://doi.org/10.1136/bmj-2023-075847

[8] Sibold, J. & Berg, K., 2010. Mood enhancement persists for up to 12 hours following aerobic exercise: A pilot study. *Perceptual and Motor*

Skills, 111(2), pp.333–342. https://doi.org/10.2466/02.06.13.15.PMS.111.5.333-342

[9] Seligman, M.E.P., 1999. Presidential address: Psychology as a half-baked cake. *American Psychologist*, 54(8), pp.559–562. Speech delivered at the 106th Annual Convention of the American Psychological Association, San Francisco, CA, August 1998. https://doi.org/10.1037/h0087671

[10] Fredrickson, B.L., 1998. What good are positive emotions? *Review of General Psychology*, 2(3), pp.300–319. https://doi.org/10.1037/1089-2680.2.3.300

[11] Hanson, R., 2020. *Velcro for the bad, Teflon for the good*. Article published on Rick Hanson's personal website, 31 January. Available at: RickHanson.com.

[12] Algoe, S.B., 2012. Find, remind, and bind: The functions of gratitude in everyday relationships. *Social and Personality Psychology Compass*, 6(6), pp.455–469. https://doi.org/10.1111/j.1751-9004.2012.00439.x

[13] Gollwitzer, P.M. & Brandstätter, V., 1997. Implementation intentions and effective goal pursuit. *Journal of Personality and Social Psychology*, 73(1), pp.186–199. https://doi.org/10.1037/0022-3514.73.1.186

www.ingramcontent.com/pod-product-compliance
Lightning Source LLC
Chambersburg PA
CBHW061230070526
44584CB00030B/4065